COGNITIVE-BEHAVIORAL THERAPY
FOR ADULT ADHD

Cognitive-Behavioral Therapy for Adult ADHD

TARGETING EXECUTIVE DYSFUNCTION

MARY V. SOLANTO

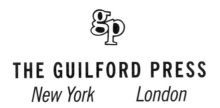

THE GUILFORD PRESS
New York   London

© 2011 The Guilford Press
A Division of Guilford Publications, Inc.
370 Seventh Avenue, Suite 1200, New York, NY 10001
www.guilford.com

Paperback edition 2013

Printed in the United States of America

This book is printed on acid-free paper.

Last digit is print number: 9   8   7

The authors have checked with sources believed to be reliable in their efforts to provide
information that is complete and generally in accord with the standards of practice that are
accepted at the time of publication. However, in view of the possibility of human error or
changes in behavioral, mental health, or medical sciences, neither the author, nor the editor and
publisher, nor any other party who has been involved in the preparation or publication of this
work warrants that the information contained herein is in every respect accurate or complete,
and they are not responsible for any errors or omissions or the results obtained from the use of
such information. Readers are encouraged to confirm the information contained in this book
with other sources.

Library of Congress Cataloging-in-Publication Data

Solanto, Mary V.
    Cognitive-behavioral therapy for adult ADHD : targeting executive dysfunction / Mary V.
    Solanto.
        p. cm.
    Includes bibliographical references and index.
    ISBN 978-1-60918-131-4 (hardcover : alk. paper)
    ISBN 978-1-4625-0963-8 (paperback : alk. paper)
    1. Attention-deficit disorder in adults. 2. Cognitive therapy. I. Title.
RC394.A85S656 2011
616.85′89—dc22
                                                                                2011003538

About the Author

Mary V. Solanto, PhD, is Clinical Associate Professor of Psychiatry in the Department of Psychiatry and at the New York University (NYU) Child Study Center at the NYU Langone Medical Center. Dr. Solanto has worked extensively with adults and children with ADHD. Her research and publications address the cognitive and behavioral functioning of individuals with ADHD, the effects of psychostimulants, and the characteristics of the subtypes of ADHD. Dr. Solanto is active in the training of psychiatrists and psychologists to diagnose and treat ADHD and related disorders. She serves on the editorial board of the *Journal of Attention Disorders* and presents to adult groups on strategies to improve organization and self-management.

About the Contributing Authors

David J. Marks, PhD, is Director of the Mount Sinai Learning and Development Center in New York City, a comprehensive faculty practice that provides neuropsychological assessments to children and adults with suspected learning and developmental disorders. Dr. Marks conducts clinical supervision in the areas of disruptive behavior disorders, pediatric neuropsychology, and psychological assessment. His rresearch activities have focused on the roles of neurocognitive and familial factors in the expression and course of ADHD, as well as the development of novel psychosocial interventions for individuals with the disorder. Dr. Marks has authored or coauthored over 20 articles and 8 book chapters, and serves as a reviewer for scientific journals in the areas of child psychology and pediatric neuropsychology.

Katherine J. Mitchell, PsyD, is a clinical psychologist in private practice, Assistant Clinical Professor at Albert Einstein College of Medicine, and Attending Psychologist in the Substance Abuse Treatment Program at Montefiore Medical Center in New York City. Dr. Mitchell has expertise in the treatment of addictions, ADHD, anxiety disorders, and PTSD, as well as the integration of cognitive-behavioral and interpersonal interventions. Previously, she served as Director of Clinical Assessment for the Collaborative Study on the Genetics of Alcoholism, a national project investigating biological correlates of substance use disorders.

Jeanette Wasserstein, PhD, ABPP-CN, is a psychologist who is board-certified in neuropsychology and has a private practice in New York City, specializing in the assessment and treatment of adults with neurodevelopmental disorders, and a member of the clinical faculty of the Mount Sinai School of Medicine. Dr. Wasserstein is the founder of the Clinical Neuropsychology Program at the New School for Social Research. She has published extensively for both the scientific and general population, including several books on learning disorders and ADHD in adults.

Contents

Purchasers of this book can download
copies of the session exercises from
www.guilford.com/solantoforms

Introduction

MARY V. SOLANTO

The treatment program described in this book evolved out of response to the clinical needs of our patients. In 1999, the Attention-Deficit/Hyperactivity Disorder (ADHD) Center at the Mount Sinai School of Medicine was inaugurated. Although the Center was initially intended primarily to address the needs of children with the condition, adults soon began to self-refer for diagnostic evaluation and treatment. Many were parents who first recognized that they themselves might have ADHD when their children were diagnosed. It soon became apparent that medication, while helpful, was in most cases not sufficient to meet the needs of these adult patients. In the pithy description of one participant, "The medication helps me focus, but it doesn't tell me what to focus *on*." These adults described long-standing problems of attentional focus, distractibility, failure to complete short- and long-term tasks and projects, disorganization, and tardiness that had persisted from childhood and had impaired their academic and occupational performance over the years, and generated considerable emotional distress. Given the pronounced difficulties in everyday executive self-management experienced by adults with ADHD, and the insufficiency of medication to address these difficulties, it became clear that a new psychosocial intervention was needed. The program developed at Mount Sinai utilizes behavioral and cognitive-behavioral methods to impart skills and strategies to enhance participants' abilities to manage time, organize, and plan in daily life. Also incorporated are traditional cognitive-behavioral interventions, as these are typically used to address problems of anxiety and depression.

1

The earliest version of the treatment program included modules to address problems of impulse and mood control, and interpersonal communication, in addition to executive self-management. However, clinical experience revealed that whereas problems of inefficiency and disorganization are virtually universal among adults with ADHD, problems of impulse control and communication are not. Furthermore, it appeared likely that a separate, equally intensive and extensive program employing different methods of intervention would be necessary to treat these problems.

The development and refinement of the cognitive-behavioral therapy (CBT) intervention was guided by the following objectives:

1. To develop a program that is sufficiently intensive and extensive to bring about *enduring* change in behavior—including development of new skills, behavioral repertoires, and adaptive cognitions to circumvent and compensate for the deficits associated with ADHD.
2. To deliver a program that is practical and can be easily incorporated into the activities of daily life in a way that becomes habitual and automatic.
3. To develop a manualized program that could be replicated and researched under controlled conditions, and disseminated to other therapists.

The group modality proved to be particularly advantageous. Common difficulties and common remedial skills and habits lend themselves to structured presentation, illustration, and practice. In addition, the group affords opportunities for modeling and vicarious reinforcement of successful strategies. Perhaps most importantly of all, the group structure provides for mutual support and encouragement among members and helps to sustain momentum toward growth and improvement. Finally, the group is a cost-effective delivery mode. Nonetheless, there are cases and clinical practices in which individual treatment is necessary or desirable and this treatment is easily modified for delivery to individuals, as described fully in Chapter 5.

In Chapter 1, I present the diagnostic criteria for ADHD, describe the typical presenting problems in adults with respect to both core symptoms and functional difficulties, and explain how the program is designed to address these problems. Accurate diagnosis is a necessary prerequisite for effective treatment. Problems of attention and/or impulsivity are common to multiple disorders and conditions, including anxiety, depression, post-traumatic stress disorder, adjustment disorder, and stress. A careful evaluation, described in Chapter 2, encompasses a review of both child and adult development and is necessary to establish or rule out ADHD and identify comorbid conditions. To illustrate the diagnostic process, we present a prototypical case of each subtype. Chapter 3 provides specific guidance for the therapist in implementing the treatment described in the Treatment Manual, including effective styles of presentation to the group, and a description of the various "hats" the effective therapist wears (teacher, cheerleader, etc.). This section also details the clinical approach to the all-important review and inquiry of the home exercise that occurs in the first part of each session. In Chapter 4, we present examples of successful treatment cases as well as more challenging types of cases, with guidance as to how the resistance may be recognized and addressed early in the treatment process. Chapter 5 describes modification of the group program to treat individuals. Chapter 6 comprises a summary of the evidence base for cognitive-behavioral approaches in general, and our program in particular, to treat adults with ADHD. The book concludes with a list of resources including software, devices, books, self-help groups, and websites.

Our goals in publishing this Treatment Manual and accompanying Therapist Guide are to share with other therapists the benefits of our clinical and research experience and to provide the tools necessary to effectively treat this common and impairing condition.

THERAPIST GUIDE

CHAPTER 1

The Adult with ADHD and the Development of the Treatment Program

MARY V. SOLANTO

Josh dashes into my office, not bothering to stop at the receptionist's desk. He is 25 minutes late for our first appointment. He breathlessly apologizes and explains that he has lost the sheet of paper on which he had written our address and so has had to "guess" where we were located—no small challenge given the eight square blocks of New York City occupied by the Mount Sinai Medical Center! He is somewhat disheveled and looks, in fact, as though he has just tumbled out of bed, but he is otherwise good-looking, with an appealing grin. Josh is a young fellow of 27, a talented writer who is enrolled in a graduate program in journalism. His primary concern right now is that he is accumulating incompletes in his graduate courses and is afraid he will be unable to complete the program by the time his scholarship runs out.

Josh reports that he has difficulty initiating and maintaining focus on his work. When seized with an idea for a story or news piece, he can rapidly write several pages of good prose. However, once the initial enthusiasm wears off or he hits a roadblock, his mind starts to wander and he may stare at the computer, surf the Web, or pace about the room, generating little output for hours at a stretch. He has particular difficulty organizing research papers. He can't seem to go about it in an orderly fashion, and has difficulty working his way systematically through references and tracking the source of the salient points he wants to incorporate. He typically jumps into writing before he has a clear thesis or argument and inevitably has to backtrack, make changes, or start over. The aversiveness of the process contributes to his procrastination. Deadlines and due dates creep up on him and he typically doesn't begin working on a paper until the night before it is due. He reports that he has had these difficulties "his whole life" (indeed he was required to withdraw from college once) and he wonders, rightly, how he will ever be able to function in the real world as a journalist.

Josh also mentions that he tends to repeatedly mislay his belongings—for example, keys, cell phone, organizer. His desks at home and at school are stacked with untidy piles of papers, with no clear space to work. He wastes much time searching for needed items.

In the second session, Josh describes problems with his girlfriend, who complains that he is impatient with her, is usually late when he is supposed to meet her, often seems not to be listening when she is talking, and forgets to do the things she asks him to do. He is also prone to get angry over "stupid little things." She has expressed surprise and concern that although he is on a budget limited by his graduate school stipend, he intermittently splurges on expensive items like a state-of-the-art sound system or tickets to an NBA game for himself and several friends. Josh is worried that these dissatisfactions will eventually cause his girlfriend to leave him—just as his previous girlfriend did.

Josh relates that a couple of years earlier, he was diagnosed as having ADHD and had a brief trial of methylphenidate (Ritalin). Although he was less distractible and able to focus for longer periods, it didn't really help him to better plan and complete his academic work in a timely fashion, and so he just stopped taking it when the prescription ran out.

Josh's case illustrates difficulties typically seen in adults with attention-deficit/hyperactivity disorder (ADHD). He has trouble with attentional focus and concentration and, particularly, with the "executive functions" of everyday life—time management, planning, and organization. These difficulties have impaired his academic performance, and, if not appropriately treated, are likely to undermine his performance on a job as well. In addition to his difficulties with attention, Josh's presentation illustrates the impulsive symptoms that accompany those related to attention in some, but not all, individuals with ADHD, as will be further explained. Impulsivity is reflected in Josh's restlessness, impatience, tendency to angry outbursts, and imprudent spending. These constitute symptoms that are particularly likely to lead to relationship discord.

Once thought to be exclusively a disorder of childhood, it is now estimated that 4% of adults have ADHD (Kessler et al., 2006). This prevalence estimate corresponds well with results from four separate longitudinal follow-up studies that, when taken together, indicate that ADHD persists to adulthood in about half of the 8% of schoolchildren in the United States who have ADHD. These longitudinal follow-up studies have furthermore extensively documented impairment in virtually every major area of functioning in adulthood in those with ADHD, including the academic, occupational, social, and emotional domains. (Barkley, Fischer, Smallish, & Fletcher, 2006; Biederman et al., 2006c; Mannuzza, Klein, Bessler, Malloy, & LaPadula, 1998; Weiss & Hechtman, 1993). Adults with ADHD complete fewer years of education, have higher rates of unemployment and underemployment, elevated rates of antisocial behavior and arrests, more driving accidents and citations, and relationship difficulties manifested in interpersonal conflict and higher rates of marital separation and divorce. In addition, adults with ADHD have higher rates of substance and alcohol abuse disorders (18%) as well as increased rates of anxiety (51%) and depression (32%; Kessler et al., 2006), and adult women with ADHD are at greater risk for eating disorders (Biederman et al., 2010). A recent study calculated the economic cost of ADHD in terms of lost productivity and reported that adults with ADHD earned $8,900–$15,400 less per annum than those with comparable education without ADHD, yielding a nationwide total cost to the economy of $77 billion (Biederman & Faraone, 2006).

DIAGNOSTIC CRITERIA AND PRESENTING PROBLEMS

The *Diagnostic and Statistical Manual of Mental Disorders* (fifth edition [DSM-5]; American Psychiatric Association, 2013) delineates the criteria for the diagnosis of ADHD (Table 1.1). (For a complete discussion and critique of DSM criteria as they apply to adults, see Barkley, Murphy, & Fischer, 2008.) Criterion A delineates the two major symptom clusters—those that reflect inattention and those that reflect hyperactivity and impulsivity—and indicates that, for adults, at least five of the nine symptoms in one or both domains must be present for diagnosis. Individuals meeting this symptom cutoff for the inattentive domain but not the hyperactive–impulsive domain are designated as having the "predominantly inattentive" presentation, whereas those who meet symptom cutoff in both domains are designated as the "combined" presentation. A "predominantly hyperactive–impulsive" presentation is also delineated. However, it appears to be largely limited to the preschool-age group (Lahey, Pelham, Loney, Lee, & Willcutt, 2005).

The other DSM-5 criteria require onset of symptoms by age 12; impairment in more than one setting (e.g., home and work or school); and reduction in social, academic, or occupational functioning. The last criterion (E) requires exclusion of patients with certain other mental conditions or whose symptoms are better accounted for by other disorders. The typical presenting problems associated with each of the two symptom clusters in adults are described in the following sections.

Inattentive Cluster

Adults with ADHD typically report distractibility and loss of focus when they engage in reading or conversations, or attend lectures or other programs, particularly those they perceive as lengthy or boring. Adults with ADHD typically have difficulty tracking time, arrive late for appointments, and experience problems completing tasks and projects in a timely fashion. Also common is difficulty initiating tasks that are routine or otherwise lacking in novelty or interest. These may include such recurring tasks as paying bills, as well as longer-term projects such as filing taxes that may as a result be delayed by many

TABLE 1.1. DSM–5 Criteria for ADHD

A. A persistent pattern of inattention and/or hyperactivity-impulsivity that interferes with functioning or development, as characterized by (1) and/or (2):

   1. **Inattention:** Six (or more) of the following symptoms have persisted for at least 6 months to a degree that is inconsistent with developmental level and that negatively impacts directly on social and academic/occupational activities:

     Note: The symptoms are not solely a manifestation of oppositional behavior, defiance, hostility, or failure to understand tasks or instructions. For older adolescents and adults (age 17 and older), at least five symptoms are required.

     a. Often fails to give close attention to details or makes careless mistakes in schoolwork, at work, or during other activities (e.g., overlooks or misses details, work is inaccurate).

     b. Often has difficulty sustaining attention in tasks or play activities (e.g., has difficulty remaining focused during lectures, conversations, or lengthy reading).

     c. Often does not seem to listen when spoken to directly (e.g., mind seems elsewhere, even in the absence of any obvious distraction).

     d. Often does not follow through on instructions and fails to finish schoolwork, chores, or duties in the workplace (e.g., starts tasks but quickly loses focus and is easily sidetracked).

     e. Often has difficulty organizing tasks and activities (e.g., difficulty managing sequential tasks; difficulty keeping materials and belongings in order; messy, disorganized work; has poor time management; fails to meet deadlines).

     f. Often avoids, dislikes, or is reluctant to engage in tasks that require sustained mental effort (e.g., schoolwork or homework; for older adolescents and adults, preparing reports, completing forms, reviewing lengthy papers).

     g. Often loses things necessary for tasks or activities (e.g., school materials, pencils, books, tools, wallets, keys, paperwork, eyeglasses, mobile telephones).

     h. Is often easily distracted by extraneous stimuli (for older adolescents and adults, may include unrelated thoughts).

     i. Is often forgetful in daily activities (e.g., doing chores, running errands; for older adolescents and adults, returning calls, paying bills, keeping appointments).

   2. **Hyperactivity and impulsivity:** Six (or more) of the following symptoms have persisted for at least 6 months to a degree that is inconsistent with developmental level and that negatively impacts directly on social and academic/occupational activities:

     Note: The symptoms are not solely a manifestation of oppositional behavior, defiance, hostility, or a failure to understand tasks or instructions. For older adolescents and adults (age 17 and older), at least five symptoms are required.

     a. Often fidgets with or taps hands or feet or squirms in seat.

     b. Often leaves seat in situations when remaining seated is expected (e.g., leaves his or her place in the classroom, in the office or other workplace, or in other situations that require remaining in place).

     c. Often runs about or climbs in situations where it is inappropriate. (**Note:** In adolescents or adults, may be limited to feeling restless.)

     d. Often unable to play or engage in leisure activities quietly.

     e. Is often "on the go," acting as if "driven by a motor" (e.g., is unable to be or uncomfortable being still for extended time, as in restaurants, meetings; may be experienced by others as being restless or difficult to keep up with).

     f. Often talks excessively.

     g. Often blurts out an answer before a question has been completed (e.g., completes people's sentences; cannot wait for turn in conversation).

     h. Often has difficulty waiting his or her turn (e.g., while waiting in line).

     i. Often interrupts or intrudes on others (e.g., butts into conversations, games, or activities; may start using other people's things without asking or receiving permission; for adolescents and adults, may intrude into or take over what others are doing).

B. Several inattentive or hyperactive-impulsive symptoms were present prior to age 12 years.

C. Several inattentive or hyperactive-impulsive symptoms are present in two or more settings (e.g., at home, school, or work; with friends or relatives; in other activities).

(cont.)

TABLE 1.1. *(cont.)*

D. There is clear evidence that the symptoms interfere with, or reduce the quality of, social, academic, or occupational functioning.

E. The symptoms do not occur exclusively during the course of schizophrenia or another psychotic disorder and are not better explained by another mental disorder (e.g., mood disorder, anxiety disorder, dissociative disorder, personality disorder, substance intoxication or withdrawal).

Specify whether:

   314.01 (F90.2) Combined presentation: If both Criterion A1 (inattention) and Criterion A2 (hyperactivity-impulsivity) are met for the past 6 months.

   314.00 (F90.0) Predominantly inattentive presentation: If Criterion A1 (inattention) is met but Criterion A2 (hyperactivity-impulsivity) is not met for the past 6 months.

   314.01 (F90.1) Predominantly hyperactive/impulsive presentation: If Criterion A2 (hyperactivity-impulsivity) is met and Criterion A1 (inattention) is not met for the past 6 months.

Specify if:

   In partial remission: When full criteria were previously met, fewer than the full criteria have been met for the past 6 months, and the symptoms still result in impairment in social, academic, or occupational functioning.

Specify current severity:

   Mild: Few, if any, symptoms in excess of those required to make the diagnosis are present, and symptoms result in no more than minor impairments in social or occupational functioning.

   Moderate: Symptoms or functional impairment between "mild" and "severe" are present.

   Severe: Many symptoms in excess of those required to make the diagnosis, or several symptoms that are particularly severe, are present, or the symptoms result in marked impairment in social or occupational functioning.

Note. Reprinted with permission from the *Diagnostic and Statistical Manual of Mental Disorders, Fifth Edition.* Copyright 2013 by the American Psychiatric Association.

weeks, months, or even years. It is not unusual, for example, for people with ADHD to have their utilities turned off or to forfeit large penalties on bills or taxes because of late payment. In one recent case, an otherwise highly competent professional got himself in a particularly tight corner with his licensing board because he had procrastinated for years on renewing his registration to practice. Paperwork required on the job may similarly be challenging for adults with ADHD. For example, a bright woman in her 30s who worked as a sales representative was talented in communicating effectively with potential customers, but she had such difficulty filling out and submitting her expense reports in an organized and timely manner that she was ultimately dismissed. In another instance, a teacher who worked effectively and imaginatively with children was repeatedly unable to plan her curricula and file her student grade reports on time. She found the effort so exhausting that she eventually sought employment in a different field.

Adults with ADHD typically struggle to keep track of personal belongings. Disorganization at home and in the office may make it difficult to locate important papers, records, and personal items, resulting in daily inefficiency and messiness. For example, a young professor's new home was so cluttered for months with unpacked movers' boxes that it was difficult to walk from one room to another. Not only did he have to repeatedly search for needed items, he was too embarrassed and ashamed to have friends over to visit, creating obstacles in his pursuit of a social life. In the workplace, disorganization can create significant difficulty as well. An otherwise competent lawyer was unable to maintain a system for organizing client files. She had a backlog of unfiled material and therefore was unable to quickly or easily determine the status of a client's case and the next court date or legal action needed. Her position was in jeopardy until another group member, who also happened to be a lawyer who had dealt successfully with this issue, came to her workplace to help her organize her files.

Adults with ADHD are quite often enthusiastic at the start of new projects—they are excited by novelty and fresh ideas. However, when the newness wears off, when challenges are encountered, or detailed follow-up work is required, they often lose interest and energy, and move on to the next new project that promises excitement. This cycle, experienced repeatedly, typically results in a string of unfinished projects, incomplete academic courses, job changes, and even abandoned relationships. One bright young woman with a degree from an Ivy League university held 10 different jobs in the 9 years following her graduation—not because she was fired, but because she couldn't decide what she really wanted to do. Everything seemed appealing at first but ultimately became boring to her. Needless to say, over the long term this process undermines and derails the identification and achievement of major academic, occupational, and personal goals.

Hyperactive–Impulsive Cluster

The core deficit underlying this domain of symptoms is an intolerance of delay—between thought and action, or between an impulse and its expression. Adults with the combined subtype of ADHD have more difficulty than others controlling impulses of many types, including desires for food, drugs or alcohol, and sex. Impaired impulse control may thus account for the increased comorbidity between ADHD and alcohol and substance abuse/dependence, and between ADHD and eating disorders. Adults with ADHD are also more likely to drive at high speed or violate other rules of the road, accounting for their having more auto accidents and citations (Barkley, Murphy, O'Connell, & Connor, 2005). An attraction to activities that involve physical risk, such as skydiving, is also a common expression of the hyperactive–impulsive dimension of symptoms in adults with ADHD.

Impulsivity may also be manifested in one's cognitive style as a propensity to jump to conclusions or to arrive at decisions with insufficient deliberation or planning. Impulsivity can affect personal decisions large and small—from taking off on a road trip without directions or a map, to changing a job or residence with insufficient consideration of the problems or consequences that might ensue. One gentleman, bemoaning his lack of career success, expressed the impact of this tendency metaphorically when he said, "I always took the first bus that came along, instead of waiting for the one that was going where I wanted to go."

Another expression of the hyperactive–impulsive domain is motor overactivity or physical restlessness, experienced by some, but not all, adults with combined-type ADHD. It is important to note here that the expression of hyperactivity–impulsivity in adults is typically quite different from its manifestation in children. That is, whereas children with combined-type ADHD may be overtly restless or fidgety, such characteristics may be less discernible to the observer of an adult with ADHD. This is because many adults report internal feelings of restlessness or may struggle to sit through a meeting, but are usually less motorically active.

As described in greater detail below, the hyperactive–impulsive cluster of symptoms may also be expressed as verbal impulsivity.

Impact on Interpersonal Relations

Manifestations of inattentiveness as well as hyperactivity–impulsivity take a toll on relationships with family, friends, employers, and coworkers. Adults who do not listen carefully appear not to care about the feelings and needs of others. Difficulty remembering or following through on commitments to others generates disappointment and conflict and may eventually undermine trust. Difficulty tolerating delay leads adults with ADHD to interrupt conversations and activities or to be overly directive or controlling in relationships. Verbal impulsivity may also be manifested as inappropriate, insensitive, or poorly timed comments, as well as excessively verbose, detailed, or digressive speech that may be off-putting to the listener. One up-and-coming young executive, for example, was dismayed to hear from her superiors that she talked too much in staff meetings and that her comments about the work of her colleagues were "too blunt." Disinhibition may also lead to inappropriate expressions of anger, or extreme expressions of affect, which similarly alienate or distress others. Personal messiness and disorganization impact negatively on others in the household, also creating stress and conflict. In this vein, the wife of a lawyer with ADHD who has a young child confided that she feels she has "two children in the house." Given the myriad ways that the symptoms of ADHD affect others, it is perhaps not surprising that adults with ADHD are more likely to be separated or divorced (Biederman et al., 2006a) and to have difficulty in social relations with friends and coworkers (Barkley et al., 2006).

INSUFFICIENCY OF MEDICATION AS A COMPREHENSIVE TREATMENT FOR ADHD

Paralleling results with children, the stimulant drugs methylphenidate (e.g., Ritalin and Concerta) and amphetamine (e.g., Adderall and Vyvanse) have been shown to be effective in reducing the core symptoms of ADHD as measured by psychiatrists' ratings of severity of DSM-IV-TR symptoms and measures of clinical global improvement. Response rates to methylphenidate are somewhat lower than those seen in children, and have ranged from 37 to 70% in controlled studies (Adler et al., 2009; Biederman et al., 2006b; Medori et al., 2008; Spencer et al., 2005). Response rates for amphetamine-based stimulants in adults are similar to those for methylphenidate (Adler et al., 2008; Spencer et al., 2001; Weisler et al., 2006). A recent meta-analysis by Faraone and Glatt (2010) reported that the overall effect size (number of standard deviation units of difference between drug and placebo) for long-acting stimulants in adults was 0.73 ("large"), with no differences between methylphenidate-based and amphetamine-based treatments. The norepinephrine reuptake inhibitor atomoxetine (Strattera) has also been shown to significantly improve symptom ratings of ADHD in adults; however, effect sizes in two large-scale studies were 0.35 and 0.40 (Michelson et al., 2003) and thus only about 55% of the average effect size reported for the long-acting stimulants described above. Atomoxetine is useful, however, when stimulants are poorly tolerated, suboptimally effective, or when there is a potential for stimulant abuse.

For a more extensive discussion of the clinical use of medication to treat ADHD in adults, the reader is referred to articles by Spencer, Wilens, and colleagues on stimulant (Spencer, Biederman, & Wilens, 2004b; Wilens, 2008) and nonstimulant (Spencer, Biederman, & Wilens, 2004a) treatment.

Although stimulant and nonstimulant drugs are effective in treating adults with ADHD, there are limitations associated with drug treatment for this disorder. First, efficacy in these studies was documented on ratings of the core symptoms of ADHD; there is little information from these studies concerning the impact of drug treatment on specific forms of functional impairment, such as disorganization or time-management difficulties. Clinical experience indicates that because of the likely lack of development of metacognitive skills in these critical areas in childhood (Douglas, 1999) drug treatment alone may not be sufficient to remediate these deficits and that some explicit skills training in these areas in adulthood may be necessary. Second, a significant subgroup (30–50%) of adults are nonresponders or adverse responders to drug treatment, which also necessitates the use of alternate interventions. Finally, since "response" in pharmacological studies typically refers to those individuals who demonstrate at least a 30% reduction in symptoms, even many of those considered to be "responders" do not achieve full remission of symptoms, leaving room and need for improvement through psychosocial intervention.

CONCEPTUALIZATIONS OF ADHD

Executive Dysfunction

The deficits in organization and efficient self-management of individuals with ADHD may be attributed, at least in part, to underlying deficits in executive functions (Barkley, 1997; Castellanos, Sonuga-Barke, Milham, & Tannock, 2006) that encompass working memory, self-inhibition, resistance to distraction, attentional shifting, organizing, planning, and self-monitoring. These deficits have been demonstrated in numerous studies on neuropsychological tests both in adults (Hervey, Epstein, & Curry, 2004) and in children (Willcutt, Doyle, Nigg, Faraone, & Pennington, 2005). Consistent with this conceptualization, structural and functional neuroimaging studies both in adults (Seidman, Valera, & Bush, 2004) and in children (Seidman, Valera, & Makris, 2005) have revealed deficits in the volume and activation of regions of the prefrontal cortex known to subserve these executive functions. Although executive dysfunction, as defined on neuropsychological tests, is not universal among individuals with ADHD (Doyle, 2006; Willcutt et al., 2005), those adults (Biederman et al., 2006d) and children (Biederman et al., 2004) who do have executive function deficits on such measures have greater occupational and academic impairment, respectively, than those who do not. Furthermore, some noted investigators have argued that children and adults with ADHD clearly exhibit executive dysfunctions in daily life even if they are not necessarily captured on the neuropsychological tests that are conventionally used to measure such deficits (Barkley & Fischer, 2010; Brown, 2008).

A complementary view of the etiology of ADHD emphasizes a fundamental deficit in inhibitory control (Barkley, Murphy, & Bush, 2001; Nigg, 2006) that encompasses abilities to inhibit or delay a prepotent cognitive or behavioral response, stop an ongoing response, and prevent interference from extraneous stimuli. According to Barkley's model, inadequate inhibitory control gives rise over the course of development to a cascade of deficits in key self-regulatory executive functions. Inadequate inhibitory control results in a proneness to respond to immediate external or internal stimuli, and is manifested cognitively as poor working memory, distractibility, failure to carry tasks through to completion, inattention to detail, and "careless" errors. Tasks that are lengthy, multistep, or inherently challenging will be particularly vulnerable to disruption. Inadequate working memory may result in difficulties in monitoring and adjusting current behavior so as to maximize timely progress toward overarching goals. Recent research provides corroborating evidence that adults (Barkley et al., 2001) as well as children (Barkley, Koplowitz, Anderson, & McMurray, 1997) with ADHD have deficits in time tracking, which may make it more difficult for them to estimate how long a task will require or how much available time has already elapsed.

Insensitivity to Reinforcement

Another conceptualization of ADHD postulates that individuals with this condition have diminished sensitivity or responsiveness to reinforcement (rewards) such that they experience particular difficulty on tasks or activities that are inherently effortful or aversive and that provide little immediate gratification. According to this theory, the behavior of individuals with ADHD is less well controlled by learned contingencies and hence is more likely to revert to the control of task-irrelevant stimuli (distracters) (Luman, Oosterlaan, & Sergeant, 2004). More frequent, more immediate, or more salient reinforcers may therefore be necessary to compensate for a postulated *elevated reward threshold* in ADHD, as first articulated by Barkley (1989) and Haenlein and Caul (1987), and tested empirically in studies reviewed by Luman et al. (2004).

Individuals with ADHD may also have a steeper *delayed reinforcement gradient*. The delayed reinforcement gradient refers to the observation, first demonstrated in animal studies (Ainslie, 1974) that there is a dropoff in the rewarding value of distant reinforcers as a function of time into the future. The result is that the more distant the reward, the less power it has to motivate behavior in the present. Research suggests that this gradient is steeper for people with ADHD, such that delayed rewards lose their reinforcing value as a function of time delay more quickly than is the case for individuals without ADHD (Aase & Sagvolden, 2006). This may explain why delayed or deferred reinforcers, such as advanced educational degrees, job promotions, and accumulated savings toward large purchases (e.g., house or car) appear to be less effective in motivating and sustaining effort toward those goals in individuals with ADHD.

Arousal and Activation

Another approach to understanding ADHD focuses on arousal and activation processes, mediated by subcortical brain regions. The former are concerned with perceptual input, whereas the latter mediates response output. These concepts were first delineated by Tucker and Williamson (1984), and were recapitulated and applied to ADHD in the "cognitive-energetic model" by Sergeant (2005). This model posits the existence of arousal and activation "pools" of cognitive resources, both of which are maintained and modulated by an overarching "effort" pool. Slow or inaccurate processing of incoming information implicates a deficit in arousal, whereas poor readiness to respond or inaccurate responding implicates a deficit in activation. A series of studies testing this model in children with ADHD, reviewed by Sergeant, found little evidence for arousal deficits but did find deficits in activation. The analogous research has not yet been conducted in adults. In the rest of this book, we shall use the term "activation" broadly to refer to self-mobilization and initiation of tasks, which many adults with ADHD find difficult.

Multiple Pathways

It should be noted here that models of ADHD based on executive dysfunction and those based on altered motivation or sensitivity to reinforcement, or cognitive-energetic factors, are not necessarily incompatible, but rather may represent alternate or combined pathways to ADHD in different individuals, capturing the heterogeneity within this diagnostic category (Sonuga-Barke, Sergeant, Nigg, & Willcutt, 2008; Sonuga-Barke, 2003).

Comorbid Anxiety and Depression

The pronounced and persistent difficulties experienced by individuals with ADHD in self-mobilization, organization, time management, and sustained effort ultimately interfere with the accomplishment of long-term educational, occupational, and personal goals. Underachievement and ineffectiveness over years, beginning in childhood and persisting through critical stages of development into adulthood, contribute to feelings of inadequacy and low self-esteem, which may ultimately lead to depression, commonly comorbid with ADHD in adults. Feelings and fears of incompetence may also give rise to performance anxiety or to obsessive and perfectionistic "compensatory" cognitions and behaviors. In addition, projection of future failures may perpetuate feelings of demoralization or depression. These negative emotions constitute further obstacles to effective self-management and must be addressed in their own right in treatment.

PROGRAM PRINCIPLES AND COMPONENTS

The program of treatment described in this book was designed to address many of the most common problems and complaints that are documented as areas of deficit for adults with ADHD and freely vocalized by patients as sources of distress and frustration: inefficiency, failure to complete tasks, difficulties initiating and terminating tasks and activities in a timely fashion, disorganization, poor planning, procrastination, tardiness, forgetfulness, indecisiveness, difficulty prioritizing, and perfectionism. In this book, treatment for ADHD comprises a set of highly structured interventions that address the multiple postulated mediators of these difficulties in ADHD that, as described above, include executive dysfunction, reduced sensitivity to reinforcement, deficits in activation, and irrational dysphorogenic cognitions. It is likely the case that these deficits are represented to different degrees in different adults with ADHD. Ultimately, with further research, we may be able to delineate these individual differences and use this information to identify a priori the subsets of skills and strategies that will most directly address each patient's needs.

The interventions may be categorized as described below and listed in Table 1.2.

Explicit Skills Training

Some treatment components may be described as training in explicit skills for self-management that, either because of attentional deficit or lack of exposure in the course of development, some adults with ADHD may never have had an opportunity to acquire. Included in this category are discussions of the mechanics of planner use to schedule and prioritize daily tasks, and the organization of physical space to maximize efficiency.

Development of Compensatory Strategies

This treatment program does not attempt to directly habilitate fundamental deficits in executive function. Rather the program aims to inculcate cognitive and behavioral

TABLE 1.2. Catalogue of Strategies/Skills to be Developed during the Cognitive–Behavioral Treatment Program

Strategies/skills	Cognitive-behavioral principle	Session(s)
Regular attendance at group	Positive habit	1
On-time attendance at group	Positive habit	1
Completion of in-home exercises	Positive habit	1
Time estimation	Explicit skill	2
Use of planner for scheduling	Explicit skill; positive habit	2
Breaking down tasks/projects into manageable parts	Compensatory strategy; self-reinforcement	3, 7, 8, 9
Contingent self-reinforcement	Contingency management	3, 7, 8, 9
Timely initiation of tasks	Self-cue and reinforcement; compensatory strategy	3, 4, 5
Timely termination of tasks	Compensatory strategy	3, 4
Use of planner for to-do lists	Explicit skill; compensatory strategy	4
Use of planner for prioritizing	Explicit skill; compensatory strategy	4
Follow-through of daily items on agenda	Stimulus management; compensatory strategy	4, 5, 6
Identifying interfering/self-sabotaging cognitions/emotions	Challenging negative self-statements	5
Visualization of long-term rewards	Self-reinforcement	6
Resistance to distractors	Compensatory strategy; anticipatory self-reinforcement	6
Organization of physical space for efficiency	Explicit skill; stimulus management; compensatory strategy	7, 8
Organization of physical space to reduce distraction	Stimulus management; compensatory strategy	7, 8
Maintenance of organizational systems	Immediate and anticipatory self-reinforcement; stimulus management	9
Planning/organization of projects	Explicit skill	10, 11
Execution of long-term projects	All enumerated principles	11
Self-instruction via maxims	Self-instructional training; self-cueing, positive habit formation	All

strategies that can compensate for deficits in executive functions, or that can induce patients to more consistently and effectively utilize the executive skills they already possess. Examples include setting up a work environment to minimize potential distracters and maximize the salience of prompts related to targeted goals, and setting a timer to cue the completion of one task or activity and transition to the next. The first is intended to compensate for poor resistance to distraction, and the second for a deficit in time tracking and/or self-inhibition.

Use of Reinforcement

The experience of reinforcement is enhanced in two ways: (1) the program incorporates strategies intended to help participants compensate for a deficit in sensitivity to reinforcement that, as described, may bear an etiological relationship to the symptoms expressed in ADHD; and (2) direct experiences of reinforcement are provided by the home exercises (and group feedback) in order to promote the acquisition, generalization, and maintenance of the behavioral and cognitive changes engendered by the program.

Compensation for Deficit in Reward Sensitivity

Just as effective behavioral interventions for children with ADHD entail increasing the frequency, salience, and immediacy of reinforcement contingent upon desired target behaviors, so too adults with ADHD are taught to schedule their activities so as to increase the frequency and intensity of experiences of reinforcement. For adults, the latter include feelings of satisfaction and experiences of competence and achievement, as well as pleasant events and other more visceral behavioral reinforcers. This is accomplished by such methods as teaching adults with ADHD to break down tasks into smaller, more manageable parts followed by breaks and/or pleasurable scheduled activities, or, when feasible, to *pair* aversive or effortful activities with pleasurable ones. In order to compensate for a steeper delayed reinforcement gradient, participants are also taught to actively visualize the future rewards that will be obtained upon completion of current effortful and/or aversive tasks (positive visualization), thereby increasing the motivational influence of those delayed reinforcers in the present moment.

Facilitation of Generalization and Maintenance

In order to facilitate the automatization of new cognitive and behavioral skills, participants are provided with simple-to-remember mantras or maxims that are introduced in the relevant session and repeated strategically throughout the program. Examples include "If it's not in the planner, it doesn't exist" and "If you're having trouble getting started, then the first step is too big." These self-instructive cognitions are designed to facilitate positive habit formation by strengthening connections between the cue (the problem situation or stimulus) and an adaptive response, thereby facilitating generalization and maintenance of the adaptive behavior in the real world.

The structure of the program is designed to increase the likelihood that participants will be reinforced for their efforts to make changes so that new behaviors will be encouraged and maintained. Toward this end, the sequence of home exercises begins with small, easy-to-manage tasks and progresses to more complex ones. In this way, exercises are designed to maximize early experiences of success and help patients to overcome their fears of failure and negative self-attributions and expectations. The roundtable review of the Take-Home Exercise allows ample opportunity for social reinforcement of positive change in the form of praise, encouragement, and support from the therapist and from other group members. In-session exercises provide further opportunities for modeling of the therapist and other group members. Throughout the program, progressive shaping of adaptive behaviors, and cognitive and behavioral rehearsal and overlearning are fostered. The ultimate goal is that the newly acquired positive behaviors and cognitions become self-reinforcing and therefore autonomously maintained.

Facilitation of Activation

Several strategies are directed toward helping participants self-mobilize to begin work on tasks that are complex or aversive. The mantra "Getting started is the hardest part" is designed to reassure and remind participants that, once they start, the going will get progressively easier. Other strategies, particularly in Session 3, are designed to facilitate the activation process by guiding participants to break down difficult tasks into manageable parts.

Identifying and Resisting Emotional Distracters

Individuals are taught to recognize and challenge the anxiogenic and depressogenic self-statements that interfere with the effective deployment of executive skills, undermine motivation and progress, and serve to maintain negative self-attributions and emotional states. The cognitive-behavioral program for addressing irrational thoughts is introduced in Session 5 and draws upon the theory and methods first introduced and applied to the treatment of anxiety and depression by Aaron Beck, Albert Ellis, and others (Butler, Chapman, Forman, & Beck, 2006). Subsequently in the program, these cognitions are identified and addressed whenever appropriate in the course of discussions during the session, particularly during the review of the Take-Home Exercise. Examples of commonly occurring irrational cognitions among adults with ADHD include the following:

Disqualifying the Positive. After completing a difficult task, the patient says to him- or herself, "I should have been able to do that a long time ago. That was nothing. Look how much more I still have to do." Rather than congratulating him- or herself and taking pride in the progress achieved, the patient undermines the value of the accomplishment. This quickly saps motivation, leading to demoralization and perpetuating the negative belief that "I can't get anything done, I am ineffective."

Perfectionism. Patients who set perfectionist standards for themselves are typically anxious about their performance and self-worth. If their product, effort, or output is not "the best" or without flaw, they are embarrassed, feel they have failed, and are reluctant to complete or submit the paper, letter, or project. The typical underlying belief here is "If it is not perfect, then it is no good at all, and I have failed." As a result of this thinking, patients may avoid or procrastinate on tasks because they are perceived as entailing insurmountable challenges.

Impact on Response to the Program. The anticipation of failure and the fear of failure are highlighted above because they may interfere with patients' deriving benefit from the very treatment program that is intended to address their difficulties. Patients who *anticipate* failure may be haphazard and uncommitted in their participation, particularly with respect to the Take-Home Exercises. The patient who *fears* failure may also avoid the Take-Home Exercises—or may do them in excessive and exhaustive detail (e.g., typing out several pages of response). Not uncommonly, anxious patients attribute their failure to use a to-do list and planner to their worry about seeing at the end of the day a list of all the things they failed to accomplish. Highlighting and helping to moderate these patients' excessive and unrealistic expectations of themselves is an important first step in facilitating a positive response to the treatment program.

The application of cognitive-behavioral interventions to treat anxiety and depression is further illustrated in the challenging treatment cases described in Chapter 4. A more detailed discussion of the application of cognitive-behavioral treatment to address dysphorogenic cognitions in adults with ADHD, which includes instructive samples of therapist–patient dialogues, may be found in *Cognitive-Behavioral Therapy for Adult ADHD: An Integrative Psychosocial and Medical Approach* (Ramsay & Rostain, 2007).

TABLE OF SKILLS AND STRATEGIES

Table 1.2 delineates the strategies and skills to be developed during the program. The session(s) during which each strategy or skill is first or primarily presented is also indicated in the table. However, it must be emphasized that the program is cumulative and reiterative, such that previously presented skills and strategies are continuously reinvoked and reapplied in new behavioral contexts, both in the sessions and in the review of the Take-Home Exercise, in order to facilitate generalization and maintenance.

Summary

ADHD persists to adulthood in a sizable percentage of children and is accompanied by significant impairment in virtually every area of adult functioning. Medication, while effective in alleviating core symptoms, is often inadequate to address these functional difficulties. Our program was developed to address critical deficits in everyday executive self-management, including time management, organization, and planning.

Good treatment begins with a good assessment. In the next chapter we describe the components of a comprehensive evaluation for ADHD, and delineate the methods whereby the primary symptoms, comorbid conditions, and associated impairments are ascertained. The chapter concludes with presentations of prototypical clinical cases illustrating the combined and predominantly inattentive subtypes.

CHAPTER 2

Diagnostic Evaluation of ADHD in Adults

MARY V. SOLANTO, DAVID J. MARKS, *and* JEANETTE WASSERSTEIN

Appropriate diagnosis is critical. If the individual is experiencing anxiety, depression, or borderline personality disorder (all of which may present with problems of attention) rather than ADHD, then the patient should be referred for interventions designed specifically to address those disorders. Of course, as described in the last chapter, anxiety and depression are often secondary to the impairments engendered by the primary symptoms of ADHD. In these cases, relief through treatment of the ADHD-related impairments may bring about relief of the secondary internalizing problems as well.

GOALS OF THE EVALUATION

ADHD can be challenging to evaluate in adults. The goals of the diagnostic assessment are multifold: (1) to ascertain whether symptoms of ADHD are currently present in sufficient scope, frequency, and severity to meet criteria for diagnosis; (2) to ascertain whether symptoms were present in childhood, as required by DSM-5 diagnostic criteria and our current understanding of this disorder; and (3) to determine what other conditions may be present—either as comorbid diagnoses or as conditions that may provide an alternate account of the symptoms that now appear to represent ADHD. The latter conditions include anxiety, depression, bipolar disorder, borderline personality disorder, substance abuse, alcohol abuse, and learning disabilities. The evaluation is complicated by the fact that all of these conditions are known to *co-occur* with ADHD at greater than expected frequencies, as described in the previous chapter. The assessment also seeks to determine the *relative urgency and priority* of current symptoms and impairment, and the implications of these for the choice of appropriate treatments and their staging. The presence of some comorbid conditions may have direct implications for the choice of treatments of ADHD—for example, comorbid substance abuse may contraindicate the use of stimulants and may indicate that treatment for substance abuse should take priority. The presence of depression or severe anxiety may indicate the need for pharmacotherapy to treat those conditions, in addition to medications for ADHD. Response to physical or emotional abuse or chronic depression in childhood can be particularly hard to differentiate retrospectively from ADHD symptoms.

OVERVIEW OF EVALUATION PROCEDURES

A comprehensive evaluation generally requires two or more interviews. The first interview typically focuses on current symptoms and impairment and begins with a review of the history. The second continues and completes the inquiry into the individual's lifetime behavioral, cognitive, emotional, social, and family functioning in order to elicit current and childhood symptoms across potential diagnoses and associated impairment. The third session is reserved for the therapist to present and explain the basis for the diagnosis or diagnoses, to discuss treatment alternatives, and to provide psychoeducation about ADHD and/or other diagnoses present.

At the outset of the evaluation, the patient is asked to complete well-normed questionnaires that establish the frequency and severity of symptoms of ADHD and of other possible comorbid conditions, including depression. When appropriate, and with the consent of the patient, a close associate (e.g., parent, sibling, friend, or partner) may be asked to complete analogous ratings. Neuropsychological testing may be useful when the results of the clinical interview are ambiguous or when other cognitive disorders, such as learning disabilities or dementia, are suspected. A structured diagnostic interview, during which the patient is asked a standardized, comprehensive set of questions about the symptoms of ADHD and/or about other DSM-5 disorders, is usually used to verify diagnoses in rigorous fashion for research purposes. However, a structured interview for ADHD, such as the Conners' Adult ADHD Diagnostic Interview for DSM-IV-TR (CAADID) (Epstein, Johnson, & Conners, 2001) may be very useful for everyday clinical applications when symptoms are ambiguous.

COMPONENTS OF THE CLINICAL INTERVIEW

The areas of inquiry to be covered by an effective clinical interview are outlined in Table 2.1 and detailed below.

TABLE 2.1. Components of the Clinical Interview

• Referral	• Medical history
• Presenting problems	• Substance/alcohol use
• History of previous psychological/ psychiatric evaluation and treatment	• Other symptoms
	• Individual interview (behavior and demeanor in the session, including mental status)
• Developmental and educational history	
• Employment history	• Questionnaires
• Family history	• Psychometric testing
• Social history	

Referral and Identifying Information

Pinpointing how the referral was initiated and processed may yield important information. When a spouse initiates the referral, for example, one must be alert to the possibility of marital dysfunction.

Presenting Problems

The primary presenting problems are important clues to diagnosis. Typical presenting complaints of adults with ADHD are described below. When the primary problem cited relates to depression or anxiety, the diagnosis may be less likely to be ADHD.

History of Previous Psychological/Psychiatric Evaluations and Treatment

The results of prior psychological or neuropsychological testing may be helpful in the current evaluation. The treatment history may provide indication of the severity, duration, and impact of symptoms of ADHD and/or comorbid conditions. Childhood psychological testing and/or treatment reports, as well as grades and qualitative comments on report cards, may help to confirm or refute a childhood history of ADHD, learning disorders, and other conditions.

Developmental and Educational History

The clinician should conduct a systematic inquiry of the individual's emotional, social, behavioral, and cognitive growth and development. This should include relationships in the family of origin, and the timing of and response to family stressors, any of which may be important to understanding the etiology of childhood emotional and behavioral symptoms.

   The educational history should include the individual's academic performance, performance on standardized tests, study skills, and deportment in elementary school, high school, and college. Typical manifestations of ADHD at each of these stages of development are described in detail below.

Employment History

The patient's quality of performance on the job can provide critical information about the nature and impact of symptoms in adulthood. The interviewer should inquire closely about current and previous job demands and performance—both as self-evaluated and as conveyed by the employer in feedback to the patient. Distinctions between performance per se (such as timeliness, accuracy, and thoroughness of completion of tasks and projects) and interpersonal relations at work may have implications for the presence of the inattentive versus hyperactive–impulsive symptom clusters, respectively, as further described below. The reasons for job changes—whether self-initiated or the result of being fired—are often revealing. The former may be related to the boredom, loss of interest, and lack of long-term direction typically experienced by adults with ADHD, whereas the latter may index the severity of impairment due to the primary symptoms.

Family History

The family history of psychiatric illness reveals the disorders for which the patient is at greatest risk. The interviewer should inquire systematically about possible ADHD, learning disabilities, depression, anxiety, and substance and alcohol abuse in the patient's biological relatives, including parents, children, siblings, and siblings' children.

Social History

The patient's social functioning and friendship patterns in childhood, high school, college, and beyond may be important in differential diagnosis and treatment planning. Children with ADHD, combined type, typically have no difficulty *making* friends because they are disinhibited and outgoing, but do have difficulty *maintaining* friendships because their unpredictable and intrusive, or aggressive behaviors alienate peers. Children with ADHD, predominantly inattentive type, by contrast, are more likely to have difficulty initiating friendships and therefore are at greater risk for peer neglect. As described in the previous chapter, ADHD often impacts negatively on the adult's interpersonal relationships.

In an adult, a history of social anxiety may offer an alternative or additional explanation for the individual's lack of satisfying social relations. A deficit in social relatedness may be consistent with Asperger syndrome or schizoid personality disorder, and these alternative diagnoses should be considered when a significant difficulty in social relations is part of the presenting clinical picture.

A persistent pattern of antisocial behavior (lying, stealing, cheating, aggression) in childhood may indicate oppositional defiant disorder or, in more severe cases, conduct disorder, both of which occur comorbidly with ADHD at higher percentages than they occur in the childhood population at large. Continuation of similar behavior in adulthood may indicate the presence of antisocial personality disorder.

Substance/Alcohol Use

It is important to inquire about past and current use of alcohol and licit and illicit drugs, given awareness that adults with ADHD are at 2.8 times greater risk of abusing drugs or alcohol than those without ADHD.

Other Symptoms

The evaluation should include systematic inquiry for symptoms other than the presenting problems, including those of anxiety, depression, and personality disorders. The clinician should be alert for the timing and sequence of onset of symptoms. When depression, for example, precedes or coincides with the onset of disorganization, shortened attention span, and reduced effort at work, these cognitive and behavioral symptoms may more likely constitute manifestations of the depression, rather than symptoms of ADHD. Yet, it is not uncommon for adults with ADHD to develop depression as a *consequence* of repeated failure experiences in the academic or occupational spheres due to ADHD-related difficulties. The same caveats hold true for anxiety, which can itself generate difficulty concentrating, initiating tasks, paying attention, and working accurately. Similarly, adults with ADHD often develop comorbid anxiety disorders because their experiences have generated self-doubt, and feelings and fears of inadequacy or rejection.

Individual Interview

Here one notes the features typically included in a mental status exam. Particularly relevant to ADHD are punctuality of arrival; dress (neatness, grooming); social appropriateness of entry and greeting behavior; rate, pitch, volume, and modulation of speech; and organization of language (e.g., digressive, well organized, verbose, provides unnecessary detail). This is also an opportunity to note signs of physical restlessness, inattention, poor working memory, and verbal impulsivity (e.g., interrupts). It is also important to observe mood and anxiety level. Eye contact and social relatedness may be relevant to a differential among ADHD, Asperger syndrome, and social anxiety disorder.

Clinical History in Childhood

It is important to obtain a history of the adult's childhood experiences in school and at home. This information will be important in determining whether the adult has ADHD, as well as identifying the source and emergence of other conditions that may be secondary to, or comorbid with, ADHD. Typical descriptions by parents and teachers of children with ADHD, irrespective of subtype, are the following: inattentive and easily distracted in class and during homework; does not perform to level of ability or performance fluctuates; exerts insufficient effort; fails to listen; fails to follow oral or written instructions; makes careless errors; is disorganized; forgets to bring homework, books, or other materials needed for school or homework; and fails to complete, or is tardy in completion of, assignments, particularly term papers and reports. It is important to be aware that, as is the case for adults, children with ADHD may be able to focus, even for seemingly long periods, on activities that are especially interesting or enjoyable for them. However, what distinguishes children with ADHD from their nonaffected counterparts is difficulty in maintaining focus and effort on academic and other tasks (e.g., practice of a musical instrument or an athletic pursuit) that are not immediately gratifying, captivating, or stimulating.

Children with ADHD, combined type, exhibit, in addition, a set of problems that relate primarily to their hyperactivity–impulsivity, including the following: disruptive, noisy, or aggressive behavior; failure to comply with school rules and regulations; and restless, fidgety, or overactive behavior. Approximately half of these children also exhibit a pattern of deliberately mean, defiant, or angry behavior that qualifies them for the additional diagnosis of oppositional defiant disorder.

Children with both the predominantly inattentive and combined subtypes of ADHD are more likely to receive lower grades, to be suspended or expelled from school, and to require special educational interventions (Faraone, Biederman, Weber, & Russell, 1998; Wolraich, Hannah, Pinnock, Baumgaertel, & Brown, 1996). It is important when reviewing the school history to ascertain whether inattentiveness and underperformance are due to ADHD, to a specific learning disability, or both. If the symptoms are due to ADHD, they are more likely to be manifested across diverse academic and social contexts, whereas the signs of a learning disorder are more likely to be displayed primarily in relation to the area of the disability—such as in reading or mathematics or other subjects or activities in which those academic skills are necessary. Complicating the differential attribution of symptoms is the comorbidity between the two disorders: approximately 25% of children with ADHD have a comorbid learning disorder (Semrud-Clikeman et al., 1992). As described in greater detail below, formal psychological and neuropsychological testing are necessary to distinguish between problems of attention, organization, memory, reading speed and comprehension, and so on that are due to ADHD and those that are attributable to a learning disorder. If a retrospective determination is made that as a child the patient's academic problems were due to a learning disorder rather than to ADHD, then, by DSM-5 criteria, the adult patient does not have ADHD.

Symptoms of ADHD—particularly inattentiveness and reduced effort or motivation—may appear similar to those of posttraumatic stress disorder (PTSD), anxiety, or depression, and may also resemble a child's response to family dysfunction, or to parental abuse or neglect. In order to differentiate among these alternatives, it is necessary to take a careful history that assesses the sequence of emergence of symptoms, and considers them, in developmental context, in relation to the events, characteristics, and functioning of the family of origin. Of great importance in this context is consideration of the parents' own psychopathology and functioning—particularly with respect to the presence of ADHD, which is highly heritable. Forty percent of children with ADHD have at least one parent who has ADHD (Barkley, 2006). Parents who themselves have ADHD often have more difficulty managing their children consistently and effectively and may be less able to serve as positive role models for the appropriate expression of emotions and behavior, and for the organization of time and materials. *Attention-Deficit/Hyperactivity Disorder: A Handbook for Diagnosis and Treatment*, now in its third edition (Barkley, 2006), is an excellent, comprehensive resource for professionals concerning the diagnosis and treatment of ADHD in children.

Academic Functioning in High School and College

A bright child may be able to perform well in elementary school despite ADHD and thereby escape identification. In other instances, parents, particularly those who are engaged and closely monitor their child's academic work, may serve as "surrogate executives" for their children and take on many of the self-structuring, self-monitoring, and organizational tasks with which the child may be having difficulty. The predominantly inattentive subtype is typically identified later than the combined type (McBurnett et al., 1999) because the inattentive symptoms are less overt and less disturbing for parents and teachers. In all of these cases, recognition of ADHD may be delayed. ADHD-related symptoms, however, are likely to become more obvious and impairing as demands for independent work, self-pacing, planning, and organization increase in the course of progression to higher educational levels. In high school and college, students with ADHD typically have difficulty getting to class on time, paying attention during lectures, taking notes, and completing larger projects such as term papers, particularly those requiring research. Lacking the structure and support they may have come to rely on at home in high school, college students may succumb to impulses to sleep late, skip class, socialize instead of study, stay up late, or use alcohol or drugs. Barkley's longitudinal follow-up study showed that adolescents with ADHD are less likely to graduate from high school, less likely to enter college, and less likely to complete college than their non-ADHD peers (Barkley et al., 2006). Many find they have to withdraw and return home after a failed semester or two.

Standardized Questionnaires

Completion of standardized self-report questionnaires is an essential component of the assessment. These measures allow the clinician to ascertain quickly and easily the presence and severity of current symptoms relative to other adults in the general population. Symptoms of ADHD, including inattention, impulsivity, and hyperactivity/restlessness, may be assessed on Conners' Adult ADHD Rating Scales (CAARS; Conners, Erhardt, & Sparrow, 1999). Accompanying manifestations of ADHD with respect to memory, organization, and other executive functions may be assessed using the Brown ADD Scales (BADDS; Brown, 1996), the Behavior Rating Inventory of Executive Function—Adult Version (BRIEF-A; Roth, Isquith, & Gioia, 2005), and the recently published Barkley Deficits in Executive Functioning Scale (BDEFS; Barkley, 2011).

An advantage of the CAARS is that patients' self-ratings are compared against normative data for adults of the same gender and age range, rather than compared against adults at large. The CAARS also includes subscales of DSM-IV-TR inattentive and hyperactive–impulsive symptoms of ADHD. In addition, the CAARS has an observer form that may be completed by a spouse, family member, or close friend who may be more sensitive to some of the patient's deficits than the patient him- or herself, particularly with respect to symptoms that affect interpersonal functioning. The BADDS, BRIEF, and BDEFS questionnaires elicit situation-specific expressions of symptoms, particularly as these relate to executive functions. The BDEFS was found to correlate more closely with impairment in adults with ADHD than did results of neuropsychological testing of executive functions (Barkley & Fisher, 2010). Questionnaires are also available to assess a childhood history of ADHD symptoms, as reported by the patient (Childhood Symptom Scale—Self-Report) or by parents or other adults (Childhood Symptom Scale—Other Report) who knew the patient as a child (Barkley & Murphy, 1998).

It is important to emphasize that ADHD questionnaires simply ascertain the patient's perceived degree of current difficulties in the domains of attention, impulsivity, hyperactivity, disorganization, executive dysfunction, and so forth compared to that experienced by adults in the population at large. They can reveal nothing about the origin of these difficulties. Indeed a study showed that patients experiencing anxiety and depression, but for whom ADHD had been ruled out, received scores in the inattentive domain on the CAARS that were as high or higher than those of patients diagnosed with ADHD (Solanto, Etefia, & Marks, 2004). This finding indicates that internalizing disorders may be associated with a degree of inattention, disorganization, and poor time management that is equivalent to that experienced by adults with ADHD. Thus, it is incumbent upon clinicians to determine the onset and chronology of these symptoms and, particularly, their relation to internalizing symptoms in order to determine whether they indicate the presence of ADHD or another disorder. Questionnaires such as the Beck Depression Inventory—Second Edition (BDI-II; Beck, Steer, & Brown, 1996) are very useful in assessing the possible presence of comorbid conditions.

Neuropsychological Testing

Neuropsychological testing may be helpful in ruling in or ruling out cognitive or learning deficits as a cause of, or an accompaniment to, problems of attention and/or impulsivity. Among these are learning disabilities, dyslexia, and dementia. In addition, neuropsychological testing may be helpful in cases in which the diagnosis is ambiguous. In such instances, the pattern of scores may serve to document deficits in attention/vigilance, working memory, processing speed, and/or short-term memory for paired associates, story details, and word lists, which are commonly (but not always), observed in cases of ADHD. The Wechsler Adult Intelligence Scale—Fourth Edition (WAIS-IV) provides indices of working memory and processing speed in addition to verbal comprehension and perceptual reasoning. Discrepancies between measures of verbal comprehension on the one hand and processing speed (lower) on the other have been found to be associated with ADHD in research with children (Solanto et al., 2007) and are often observed in adults with ADHD as well (Brown, Reichel, & Quinlan, 2009). Impairments in short-term memory relative to intelligence can be identified using the verbal and nonverbal tests of the Wechsler Memory Scale (WMS; Quinlan & Brown, 2003). The Continuous Performance Test (CPT) provides a standardized assessment of attention (vigilance) as well as bias to respond (an index of impulsivity). Several CPTs with norms for adults are available commercially, including the Conners' CPT (Conners, 1994), the Integrated Visual and Auditory CPT Plus (IVA+Plus; Sanford & Turner, 2004), and the Test of Visual Attention (TOVA; Leark, Greenberg, Kindschi, Dupuy, & Hughes, 2007). These CPTs vary with respect to their relative sensitivity to inattentive versus impulsive errors, and also with respect to availability of an auditory as well as a visual modality of testing. A comprehensive review of the strengths and weaknesses of CPTs as used with adults with ADHD can be found in a review by Riccio and Reynolds (2001). Hervey and Epstein (2004) authored a comprehensive review and meta-analysis of the specificity and sensitivity of the CPT and other commonly used neuropsychological measures in identifying cases of ADHD in adults. These and other more recent findings are discussed extensively elsewhere (Wasserstein, Wolf, Solanto, Marks, & Simkowitz, 2008).

The *style* of responding during testing may provide additional information to help to establish primary or comorbid diagnoses. An impulsive response style that favors speed over accuracy and/or tends to overlook details may indicate ADHD. By contrast, a response style characterized by suboptimal effort across test domains suggests the presence of depression. Excessive concern about performance, lack of confidence in responses, and obsessive concern for details typically indicate anxiety. Anxiety may be observed to specifically interfere with performance on tasks that demand focal attention and concentration, such as arithmetic and memory tasks, as well as timed performance tests, and may thus offer an alternative, or in some cases, an additional mechanism of attentional deficits.

Questions as to whether they have a learning disability (LD) or ADHD are often the triggers for evaluation in previously undiagnosed adults (see discussion in Wasserstein & Denckla, 2009). Studies performed in children with ADHD are generally consistent in showing an elevated base rate of dyslexia and arithmetic disorders in this population (Semrud-Clikeman et al., 1992). However, there is disagreement as to the appropriateness of recognizing other types of LD, including nonverbal LD and disorders of executive dysfunction, both of which may be especially prevalent in ADHD (see Wasserstein & Denckla, 2009, for review). No studies to date have looked at the actual prevalence of learning disorders among adults with ADHD. Nevertheless, existing data from both children and adults with ADHD clearly argue that LD is highly comorbid, and thus should be formally evaluated if the clinical presentation suggests it. In this regard, questions about past school failure, requests for educational guidance, and the need for accommodations in classes and during standardized testing are especially relevant.

In older patients there may be a need to distinguish cognitive and/or attentional deficits from Alzheimer's, which also affects prefrontal, executive functions. The age at onset of symptoms will usually provide an important clue.

PROTOTYPICAL CASES OF ADHD

In this section, we present clinical case material to illustrate the process of clinical data gathering and integration for purposes of case formulation and diagnosis.

The following cases are "classic" in that (1) the primary complaints and symptoms are prototypical of ADHD; (2) there is clear evidence of impairing ADHD symptoms in childhood; (3) the frequency and severity of current symptoms are confirmed on standardized measures of ADHD; (4) there is little comorbidity to cloud or confound the clinical picture; and (5) other typical accompanying features, such as family history of ADHD, are also present. In all the cases, identifying information has been changed.

Combined Type: Beth

Referral and Presenting Problems

Beth is a 26-year-old single young woman who has her own business as a DJ and party planner. She presented herself for evaluation after having tried her friend's stimulant medication and finding it very helpful while she was planning a project.

Beth reports difficulty organizing her business—for example, she has no business plan, has conducted her business without regard for regulations or taxes she may owe, and so on. She has been unable to keep track of her income and expenses, doesn't maintain receipts or checkbook records, and doesn't pay her own bills on time. She has difficulty with the detailed planning, monitoring, and follow-up her business requires. She doesn't regularly use strategies (e.g., planner/organizer) to keep track of her schedule and is often late for appointments or misses them entirely. She often has difficulty listening attentively to her clients, and may forget what she has been told. In conversations, she is easily distracted, and may "zone out" during long presentations. She reports problems of short-term memory (e.g., goes to a store and doesn't remember what she went to buy), and has trouble planning simple sequences (e.g., errands).

Also noted are problems of impulse control and restlessness: Beth tends to get angry when delayed (e.g., in traffic); becomes restless and bored during long movies, concerts, and lectures and wants to leave; and becomes impatient while listening to others and may interrupt. When angry, she may say things she doesn't mean. Angry outbursts occur approximately three times per week, primarily with her boyfriend or best friend, after which she is extremely remorseful.

History of Previous Evaluation and Treatment

Beth has no previous evaluation and treatment history.

Developmental and Educational History

In elementary school Beth received generally average grades, but her teachers described her as "having a lot of unfulfilled potential" and "very bright but lazy." She was suspended for 1 week in first grade for hitting another child with a lunchbox and reports other similar episodes of aggression as a child for which she was frequently sent to the principal's office. She had frequent "careless" accidents, often due to tripping while rushing. In high school, she had difficulty paying attention in lectures, and frequently didn't complete homework assignments even though she found them easy. She often skipped class to be with her friends. In college, Beth had difficulty getting to class on time, and completed term papers and projects only at the last minute. She got very good grades (A's) in subjects she liked, and C's or worse in subjects she found "boring." She says she has never been good at math, which, at present, negatively impacts the financial management of her business.

Employment History

After graduating from college, Beth held a series of short-term jobs—as waitress, receptionist, and secretary—to pay the bills while she searched for "what she really wanted to do." She was dismissed from a secretarial position because of chronic lateness, and failure to complete work by deadlines.

Family History

Beth has a very supportive, close-knit family. There is a history of probable ADHD in her mother and brother. No other psychopathology is reported among family members.

Social History

Beth reports that friends may get annoyed with her for not being on time to engagements, as described above. Despite the social impact of her symptoms, Beth seems to have enjoyed good friendships during her school days, a pattern that has continued to the present.

Medical History

Beth has no significant current or past medical history.

Substance/Alcohol Use

Beth has no current or past history of excessive or inappropriate use of alcohol or substances.

Other Symptoms

Beth denied current depression during the clinical interview, but received a score of 28 (moderate) on the Beck Depression Inventory as a result of endorsing moderate levels ("2") of self-criticism, indecisiveness, worthlessness, lack of energy, early morning awakening, and disappointment in herself. Sadness was not endorsed. Some endorsed symptoms (e.g., concentration difficulty, loss of interest) may relate to ADHD symptoms.

Beth reports feeling overwhelmed by anxiety and prone to "catastrophize" about all she has to do. She worries she will lose her business because she will be unable to pay her taxes.

Individual Interview

Beth presented as an attractive, animated young woman who maintained good eye contact, and was candid, articulate, and well related. Mood was euthymic, with full range. During the feedback session she became tearful when describing the impairment and distress caused by her ADHD symptoms.

Questionnaire Results

Psychometric test results on the BADDS and CAARS—Self Report showed elevations (greater than two standard deviations above the mean) on all scales—including those measuring symptoms of inattention and hyperactivity–impulsivity, as well as features of executive dysfunction. The total T-score on the BADDS was 86 ("ADD highly probable").

Summary and Formulation

Current symptoms, developmental history, and questionnaire results all converge to yield a clear diagnosis of ADHD, combined type. Significant and pervasive difficulties are reported with respect to sustained attention, executive functions, and tolerance for delay. Beth's ADHD symptoms resulted in impairment in academic functioning and currently cause impairment and distress with respect to the management of her business and interpersonal functioning. There is a recent history of anxiety and depression due to feeling overwhelmed and inadequate. Strengths for Beth include the close and supportive relationships she maintains with her friends and family members.

Recommendations

1.   A trial of stimulant medication for management of ADHD symptoms is recommended.

2.   Individual psychotherapy is recommended in order to provide support and psychoeducation about ADHD; address problems of time management, planning, and anger management (preferably using cognitive-behavioral methods); and mitigate anxiety and depression, as described above.

3.   Neuropsychological testing to assess a possible learning disorder in mathematics.

Commentary

Beth's is a protypical case of ADHD, combined type. Although her disorder was never previously diagnosed, a review of this young woman's developmental history reveals all three of the classic symptoms—inattention, hyperactivity, and impulsivity—beginning in grade school and continuing through to the present. Inattention and disorganization currently greatly impede the efficiency of Beth's business operation. Hyperactivity–impulsivity is manifested in her low tolerance for delay, restlessness in sedentary pursuits, and angry outbursts. Despite a strong social support network, Beth reports feelings of self-criticism and worthlessness, as well as anxiety about not being able to accomplish everything she has to do, all of which are commonly experienced by adults with ADHD. Research has indicated that females with ADHD have a stronger family history of ADHD (Smalley et al., 2000) and indeed, there are two other family members who are also suspected of having ADHD in Beth's family of origin.

Predominantly Inattentive Type: Charles

The hallmark of the predominantly inattentive subtype is that the primary problems are in the area of attention—including focused and sustained attention, time management, organization, and working memory. Thus problems are primarily manifested in the domains of listening, completing work on time, and concentrating on detailed work. Contrasting with the combined type, there is a *relative absence* of problems that reflect poor impulse control, such as problems with anger management, excessive use of drugs or alcohol, overeating, imprudent sexual activity, excessive spending or financial risk taking, impulsive decision making, and physical risk taking in sports ventures.

When evaluating a potential case of ADHD, predominantly inattentive type, in an adult, it is important to rule out depression and anxiety as these disorders can cause symptoms very similar to those that are typical of the inattentive subtype. Ascertaining that at least some of the ADHD-like symptoms were present in childhood is critical to establishing their primacy. The inattentive subtype typically has a later age of onset (Applegate et al., 1997) than the combined subtype and many cases may not experience significant impairment until age 11 (McBurnett et al., 1999). Note, however, that symptoms of hyperactivity–impulsivity may have been present in childhood even when they are not salient in the current clinical picture, as recent data suggests that a substantial percentage of childhood combined-type cases convert to the inattentive type by adulthood (Biederman, Mick, & Faraone, 2000). When both ADHD-like and internalizing symptoms are present in adulthood, ascertaining their relative time of onset is critical to determining their causal relationship and thus in arriving at the correct primary and secondary or comorbid diagnosis(es) and an appropriate and comprehensive treatment plan. In the absence of the "telltale" symptoms of hyperactivity and restlessness, it may be more difficult to differentiate ADHD from learning disorders and formal testing may be needed to evaluate this alternative—or additional—diagnosis.

Referral and Presenting Problems

Charles is a 40-year-old lawyer who lives with his wife and two young children. He sought help for problems relating to procrastination, finishing tasks, prioritizing, and avoiding distractions. He has difficulty transitioning between tasks and may "fixate," spending too much time on one task to the exclusion of other more pressing demands. He also may lose focus during conversations and his mind can just "go" during meetings. He conveyed significant distress about the impact of these difficulties on his work, along with the persistent feeling that he would have gone further in his professional life had he not had ADHD-related difficulties.

At home Charles has trouble keeping track of personal finances, including budgeting, decision making, and paying bills on time; these are exacerbated by the fact that current anxieties about his financial state make it "painful" to even begin work on this. Some of these tasks (e.g., bill paying) fall to his wife, who is feeling burdened by these additional demands. He also reports a history of problems related to short temper with his wife, which now appear to be ameliorated by medication.

History of Previous Psychological/Psychiatric Evaluation and Treatment

Charles reports a history, dating back to college, of anxiety attacks that occurred unpredictably and were accompanied by feelings of nausea and "total disconnection." They remitted while in college but returned at age 30, at which time he was diagnosed with depression and obsessive–compulsive disorder (OCD) that were treated with medication, with benefit. He has not had any anxiety attacks since starting on a selective serotonin reuptake inhibitor (SSRI) 3 years ago.

Developmental and Educational History

Charles's father was a physician and his mother was a nurse. He recalls that his difficulties in school did not begin until fifth grade, when, at age 10, he became more distractible and forgetful, having difficulties with listening, sustained attention, follow-through, and organization. At a private high school, previously attended by his father, he struggled through his classes, achieving only average grades, and was told he "wasn't working up to his potential," much to the chagrin and disappointment of his parents. His problems affected his reading, writing, and arithmetic; however, inquiry suggested that he had no primary comprehension or processing difficulties in these areas. He "hit bottom" at about 17 years of age with respect to his academic struggles and consequent distress and anxiety.

After graduating from high school, Charles enrolled at a small liberal arts college, where he experienced continued difficulties in completing work and achieving expected levels academically, but he received his BA in 4 years. Thinking at first that he wanted to go into business, he completed an MBA, but found himself unchallenged and "uninspired" by his first two jobs in business consulting. He decided to switch to law and pursued his degree in night school.

Family History

Charles's son (age 6) has also been diagnosed with ADHD. Charles thinks his father may have had it as well, but the father was never evaluated or treated for the condition.

Social History

Charles tended to be somewhat shy and reserved as a child. However, he made several close friends in high school and in college, which he retains to the present day.

Medical History

Charles has no significant current or past medical history.

Substance/Alcohol Use

Charles has no current or past history of excessive or inappropriate use of alcohol or substances.

Other Symptoms

Charles reports that he worries on a nearly daily basis about getting things done and reports significant concern about generating sufficient income to finance his children's education. He feels that his worries are rational under the circumstances.

Individual Interview

Charles presented as a well-dressed, polite gentleman. He was affable and well related in the sessions and was candid and articulate in describing his difficulties. Mood appeared mildly depressed.

Questionnaire Results

Psychometric test results showed elevations (greater than two standard deviations [SD] above the mean) on the inattention/memory and DSM-IV-TR inattentive scales on the CAARS, but no elevations on scales measuring hyperactive or impulsive symptoms. On the BADDS, scales measuring activation and effort were elevated at least 1.5 SD above the mean, but scales measuring attention, affect, and memory were not. Screening on the WAIS-IV revealed scores in the superior range on both verbal and nonverbal subtests, yielding a Full Scale IQ of 140.

Summary and Formulation

Charles presents with difficulties initiating and maintaining attentional focus (both on his work and in conversation), managing time effectively, prioritizing, and planning. These difficulties are long-standing (onset at age 10), they have impaired his academic performance, and they have continued to exact a significant toll on his occupational functioning and advancement. This has generated considerable anxiety and depression (now partially improved with medication), particularly about the state of the family's finances, which in turn has exacerbated Charles's difficulty with tasks such as bill paying. The "spill over" of such tasks to his wife's responsibility has created strains in their relationship.

Recommendations

1. Trial of stimulant medication. If trials of both methylphenidate and d-amphetamine prove to be suboptimal with respect to either efficacy or side effects, then a trial of the nonstimulant Strattera (atomoxetine) should be considered.

2. Individual therapy, utilizing cognitive-behavioral techniques in order to:

a. Foster development of effective self-management strategies in time management and organization.
b. Provide support and cognitive-behavioral intervention to address anxiety and depression, which here appear to be in part secondary to the impairments generated by ADHD.

Commentary

Charles's is a prototypical case of the inattentive subtype in that his difficulties are currently and by history predominantly inattentive in nature, without the behavioral acting out that is often prominent in the profile of the combined subtype. Nonetheless one does pick up a history of difficulty related to control of temper with his wife, which serves as a reminder that patients with this subtype are not necessarily completely without symptoms in the hyperactive–impulsive domain. Description of Charles's academic struggles initially appeared so prominent as to suggest the possibility of a learning disorder. However, the lack of reported specific comprehension difficulties in math or reading and the superior WAIS-IV results in both verbal and nonverbal domains provided little support for this hypothesis. A salient feature of this case is the pronounced anxiety and the assault on self-esteem that has plagued Charles since his high school days as a result of his failure to perform to the level expected by his parents and teachers.

SUMMARY

A comprehensive evaluation for ADHD in adults includes a systematic review of symptoms and functional impairment in all domains in childhood as well as in adulthood, in addition to family history and completion of standardized self-report questionnaires.

The next chapter is a detailed "how-to" guide for therapists administering the treatment described in the Treatment Manual.

CHAPTER 3

How to Be a Successful Therapist

A Guide to Substance and Style

MARY V. SOLANTO, DAVID J. MARKS, *and* JEANETTE WASSERSTEIN

STRUCTURE AND FORMAT OF THE TREATMENT MANUAL

Please note that this material is also printed at the start of the Treatment Manual proper, as a convenience to the user. The Treatment Manual is a session-by-session guide to a 12-session treatment program designed to foster the development of time-management, organizational, and planning skills in adults with ADHD. Most sessions have Leader Notes, as well as Take-Home Notes and a Take-Home Exercise to be distributed to the participants.

The Leader Notes are intended to highlight the principles and strategies to be presented and discussed at each meeting. They are not intended to be delivered strictly as a script but rather to provide an outline of the material to be covered, along with suggested phrasing of material for greatest clarity and maximum impact upon group participants. Material that is important for the therapist to specifically articulate is presented in **bold *and italics*** and may be given verbatim. In general, however, the style of the group should remain interactive rather than expository during the presentation portion, as well as during the review of the Take-Home Exercise. Thus, group participants may pose questions or raise issues during the presentation to which the therapist may respond by using them as opportunities to explain the concepts and strategies planned for the session.

The Take-Home Notes are intended to provide a pithy review, recapitulation, and reemphasis of the material covered in the session. In some cases, additional suggestions are provided that may not have been covered in the sessions. The Take-Home Notes are intended to compensate for possible lapses of attention in the session and also to set the stage for the Take-Home Exercise. They provide a valuable tool for future reference and review and should be sent out to individuals who miss the session. An optional, but helpful, tactic is to send out an e-mail to all members midway between sessions to bolster motivation and encourage completion of the Take-Home Exercises.

FORMAT OF CBT GROUP SESSIONS

This CBT program is designed for a group of six to eight adults meeting weekly for 2 hours over 12 weeks. Our groups are scheduled in the evening, 6:30 to 8:30, so as to allow working adults to complete the workday, have dinner, and travel to the session. The format of each group session is as follows:

1. Review of Take-Home Exercise (up to 1 hour).
2. Presentation and discussion of new material (45 minutes, including In-Session Exercise).
3. In-Session Exercise.
4. Presentation and discussion of next Take-Home Exercise (15 minutes).

As described at the beginning of Session 5, the program may be expanded by including an additional session on cognitive-behavioral methods to overcome anxiety and depression. An optional additional module concerning "Getting to Bed, Getting Up, and Getting to Work on Time" is also included at the end of the Treatment Manual.

SELECTION OF CANDIDATES FOR THE CBT GROUP PROGRAM

We recommend enrolling only those individuals who have been previously diagnosed by an experienced mental health professional as having ADHD. If individuals have not been diagnosed in our own program, we require confirmation of the diagnosis in a report or direct phone conference with the diagnosing professional. We also schedule an individual consultation with every potential group member in order to confirm the usefulness and appropriateness of group participation.

As will be further discussed in Chapter 5, CBT group intervention is generally not suitable for patients with severe depression and/or suicidality or patients with borderline personality disorder because the accompanying psychopathology is too severe to be addressed or monitored in the group. In addition, patients with active alcohol or substance abuse are not suitable because they are unlikely to be able to effectively implement or, ultimately, assimilate the cognitive strategies outside the group sessions. We have also found that the group modality is not appropriate for patients who have significant difficulties in anger management because their behavior may antagonize or alienate other group members. Nonetheless, we have found that the majority of patients with ADHD who present with problems of executive self-management are good candidates for group CBT. Adaptation of the program for individual therapy is described in Chapter 5.

THERAPIST STYLE

Group therapy sessions must accomplish the following: First, the program must capture and maintain the interest of the participants who, by definition, have difficulty paying attention. Second, it must offer opportunities in the session for the participants to learn about and then begin to work through, practice, and, ultimately, assimilate the executive self-management strategies that are being imparted. Finally, it must allow for support, sharing, and mutual learning between and among participants and therapist.

To be most effective, therapists should have the following types of background: They should, first of all, have a detailed knowledge of the kinds of difficulties in everyday life that are experienced by adults with ADHD and must understand how these problems proceed from several postulated core neuropsychological deficits. They must be able to distinguish between problems of living due to ADHD and those that are due to comorbid conditions such as anxiety, depression, and reading and/or other learning difficulties. They must understand, in terms of behavioral and cognitive-behavioral principles, how the components of the program address those problems and induce the formation of new, more adaptive habits. Therapists play the following roles:

• **The therapist must be an enthusiastic cheerleader.** She should arouse hope that change is possible, who reinforces positive change when it occurs, and who maintains hope for continued improvement despite setbacks. It is important that patients be reinforced for effort, and not just success, and that both therapist and patient recognize that improvement will occur in "successive approximations" to the desired outcome.

• **The therapist must be a good teacher.** Clinicians must have a style of presentation that is clear, lively, and engaging. Comfort with showmanship is an asset here in that the therapist leads, in part, by exhortation—that is, by convincing participants, directly or indirectly, that they have the ability to change, and that practicing the strategies imparted, beginning with the Take-Home Exercises, will lead to greater comfort, satisfaction, and control in the activities of daily life. A seminar style of teaching, using the Socratic method of engaging and leading the participants through guided questioning, is most effective. Wherever possible, examples and illustrations should be sought by drawing upon the problems and experiences of the group members. Liberal use of the chalkboard or whiteboard to list, emphasize, or diagram relationships among concepts helps to focus and maintain participants' attention.

- **In general, he or she must be a good therapist.** The usual clinical expertise and sensitivity is required, of course, but is especially important when working with adults with ADHD in a group setting. Therapists should have sufficient experience in individual modalities of clinical work that they have a well-honed clinical intuitive sense of when to intervene to probe or challenge a participant's defenses, when to wait, or, in the case of group therapy, when to turn the matter over to the group and let another participant make the first observation. They must be able to gently but firmly hold the participants accountable for putting forth their best effort in completing the home exercises and applying the strategies learned.

Thus, ideally, the therapist will have experience in cognitive-behavioral treatment modalities with adults as these have been traditionally used to address anxiety and depression, as well as experience in individual and group therapy modalities with adults. Experience in the diagnostic assessment of adults with ADHD and a working knowledge of the neuropsychology of the condition are essential. Clinical experience in the diagnosis of and treatment with children with ADHD is helpful in that it gives the therapist additional insights into the ways that having ADHD impact the child and family.

USE OF THE MANTRAS

Among the challenges of working with adults with ADHD is the need to mobilize them to *utilize* the relevant strategies in everyday life. In order to facilitate this, the program, as described, makes use of maxims or "mantras," which are set off between dashed horizontal lines in the Treatment Manual. Among these are "If it's not in the planner, it doesn't exist" (cues planner use) and "A place for everything—and everything in its place" (cues strategies for set-up and maintenance of organizational systems). It is important that these be repeated liberally to the group when appropriate in order that the habits they describe become second nature. Note that it is necessary to be somewhat more didactic in this respect than one might otherwise be in working with adults. This is because many of these skills and habits are, in general, not arbitrary or "negotiable," and the individual with ADHD needs a nonambiguous statement that has clear implications for action. A complete listing of the mantras is found in Table 3.1.

In order to encourage the use of strategies in everyday life, several of the mantras incorporate a cognitive signal or cue that will remind the patient to use the strategy. Some of the mantras have the cue built into them, as in "If you're having trouble getting started, then the first step is too big." The first part of the mantra identifies the problem situation (difficulty with activation) and the second part provides the solution (break down the task into manageable parts). Similarly, the home exercises are formulated so

TABLE 3.1. List of Mantras (Maxims) Employed in the Program

1. "If it's not in the planner, it doesn't exist."
2. "If you're having trouble getting started, then the first step is too big."
3. "Do all things in the order of priority."
4. "Getting started is the hardest part."
5. "A place for everything—and everything in its place."
6. "Out of sight, out of mind."
7. "What you don't do today won't go away—it will just be that much *harder* tomorrow."

that the strategies can be easily incorporated into daily life. For example, in the session on "automatic thoughts" (Session 5), participants are asked to identify a situation in which they are aware of avoiding taking action on a task, or are feeling anxious or depressed about confronting a task. The participants are then asked to tune into the automatic thoughts they may be experiencing and to identify irrationalities. If the exercise is successful, it will encourage the participant to similarly self-examine when he or she is aware of procrastinating or of feeling anxious or depressed.

REVIEW OF THE TAKE-HOME EXERCISE

Fully half of each session is devoted to a review of the Take-Home Exercise because of its documented critical importance in effectuating lasting behavior change. It also affords the therapist an early opportunity to identify and address individual obstacles to change that are most apt to first manifest as difficulty completing the Take-Home Exercise. The therapist, therefore, should maintain an easily consulted record for each individual of whether the Take-Home Exercise for each session was completed fully, partially, or not at all.

In reviewing the Take-Home Exercises, the therapist should also be sure that participants understand that once a new strategy (e.g., prioritizing and scheduling a week's tasks) is introduced, participants should add that strategy to their personal repertoire and continue to implement it. Thus, the strategies introduced in the sessions and practiced via the Take-Home Exercises are intended to be cumulative.

During the roundtable review, each participant is asked in turn to share his or her experience in attempting to complete the Take-Home Exercise. If the exercise was completed successfully, it is important for the therapist to reinforce the success through sincere praise and to highlight and solidify the progress made by (1) asking the participant how it felt to complete the task, (2) asking what allowed the participant to be successful in accomplishing the task this time (as opposed to previous instances when he or she was not successful, and (3) asking what the participant would do again in the future when confronting a similar task or problem.

If the participant had difficulty completing the task, the therapist must systematically query the participant in order to ascertain the source of the problem and suggest an adjusted approach. The therapist should in this instance reinvoke the relevant strategies (that have been covered in the program thus far) and discuss how they might have been applied in this situation. Relevant questions might be "Did you schedule it in your planner?"; "Are you trying to do too much?"; "Did you break it down into parts?"; "Did you plan to reward yourself afterward?"; and "Were you trying to work in a space with distractions?" Sometimes participants will state as a reason for their noncompletion of the Take-Home Exercise that they are not having difficulty in the topic area covered by the exercise. Occasionally, this is genuine—for example, some individuals have difficulty in time management but not in organization. On the other hand, this denial may represent an excuse not to do the task—for example, due to anxiety or fear of failure. In either instance, the therapist might help the participant restate or refocus on his or her personal goals for the program, and, taking these into account, help tailor or modify the Take-Home Exercise for the client to address those specific needs or problems.

If no attempt was made to complete the exercise, the therapist must query the reason. If there was a crisis, sickness, or unusual burden or other interfering circumstance during the week, the therapist should, of course, empathize but encourage the participant to try to make up the exercise in the coming week, and perhaps assist in identifying opportunities when this will be most feasible. However, the therapist must be alert for a pattern of noncompletion of the Take-Home Exercise. Failure to complete two Take-Home Exercises in a row, without extenuating circumstances, often indicates the presence of oppositionality, denial, anxiety, or depression, as further illustrated in the cases presented in the next chapter. Given the demonstrated importance of the Take-Home Exercise to the overall benefit derived from the program (Chapter 6), it is important to identify and address these issues as early as possible.

Participants who are oppositional or in denial may openly question the relevance or utility of the exercise. In this context, it may be helpful to review with the participant his or her initial goals upon joining the group, explaining in this context the relevance of the exercise. Another useful approach is to help the participant to conduct a simple cost–benefit analysis of his or her typical behavior versus the new approach prescribed in the Take-Home Exercise—for example, depending on one's memory for appointments versus regularly using and checking a planner.

The anxious participant may fear being overwhelmed by or otherwise unable to complete the task, citing past failure experiences. Not uncommonly, for example, anxious participants cite fear of scheduling tasks in a planner because this overt commitment will make their subsequent failure to complete those tasks much more obvious. In this instance, it is helpful to remind participants that anxiety is common when attempting behavior change, but that they should endeavor to "push through" the anxiety and schedule tasks anyway, with the reassurance that the anxiety will diminish over time as they learn new strategies that will help them experience success in task completion.

The depressed participant is a victim of demoralization and what Martin Seligman termed "learned helplessness" (Seligman, 1975). His experience has taught him that his efforts, or he himself, will never be good enough. In describing their experiences with the Take-Home Exercises, participants with this proclivity will typically criticize themselves for whatever they didn't accomplish rather than reinforcing themselves for what they did achieve. The therapist may usefully highlight this tendency and describe how it is likely to quickly undermine further motivation and effort.

During sessions in the second half of the treatment program (i.e., after the material on automatic thoughts has been presented) it may be appropriate for the therapist to highlight how the participant's thoughts, statements, or behavior may reflect one of the "automatic thoughts" or cognitive distortions previously discussed in the program. Sensitivity to the patient's feelings and to his or her readiness to process this feedback is, of course, essential. Often, as intimacy develops among the group members, another participant may take the initiative to provide feedback. It is desirable for the therapist to let other members "say it first" since participants are often less defensive about comments received from peers in the group rather than from the therapist.

Instances of participants' avoidance of the Take-Home Exercise provide a stimulus to the therapist to reiterate, as appropriate, to the group as a whole the demonstrated value of the Take-Home Exercise for progress in the treatment program. The therapist should encourage participants to at least try the exercise, or do a part of it, on the premise that completing even a small part is "a thousand times better" than doing none at all. The therapist should also warn participants against succumbing to the temptation, born of shame, to skip the session if they have not completed the Take-Home Exercise.

A final note to the therapist is that it is important to strictly limit the discussion of the Take-Home Exercise to the first hour in order to allow enough time for presentation and discussion of the new material for the session. Many adults with ADHD are extremely talkative and may have difficulty limiting their remarks in the roundtable review. It may be helpful for the therapist to make an announcement at the outset (of the program or session) that the time allowed to each person will of necessity be limited to 8–9 minutes in order to allow time for everyone to participate, and to gently remind any one participant as necessary. In some cases where there are several very talkative participants, it may even be necessary to use a minute timer.

PRESENTATION OF THE NEXT TAKE-HOME EXERCISE

After reviewing the requirements of the next Take-Home Exercise at the end of the session, as described on the handout, it's important to have the participants begin to think about how they will approach the exercise, what problem situation or task they will apply it to, and what problems they might anticipate in trying to accomplish it so that these can be addressed in advance.

USE OF MEDICATION CONCURRENT WITH CBT

Patients may enter CBT with or without concurrent treatment with ADHD medications. On average, about half of the patients in our groups are receiving such medication. Although clinical intuition suggests that patients may be better able to attend to the material in sessions, and to more consistently apply the strategies at home while receiving concurrent treatment with stimulants or atomoxetine, our preliminary research on the subject has not shown this to be the case (see Chapter 6).

SUMMARY

In the foregoing we have provided guidance for the CBT group therapist on matters related to both substance and style. In clinical work, case examples provide an important vehicle for learning. In the next chapter, we present case studies that illustrate patients who responded easily and well to group treatment, and others who posed clinical challenges of various types.

CHAPTER 4

Profiles of Patient Response to the Treatment

Tailoring Therapy to Individual Cases

MARY V. SOLANTO, DAVID J. MARKS, JEANETTE WASSERSTEIN,
and KATHERINE J. MITCHELL

One of the advantages of the approach described herein is that it enables the therapist to ascertain fairly quickly the emotional or cognitive obstacles that are likely to impede the patient's progress in this structured treatment. In providing the CBT group sessions, we have found that there are several "types" or profiles of patients that may be identified early in the course of the group—sometimes after only one or a few sessions. Early awareness of these profiles allows the therapist to tailor the intervention to the individual needs of these patients.

Early clues to patient response are to be found in how the patient describes his or her difficulties at the outset (candid, or denies or minimizes), degree of confidence that the treatment will help, extent of participation in the group (shy and withdrawn, or open), and response to feedback from the therapist or other group members (defensive or receptive). Perhaps most revealing is the patient's response to the Take-Home Exercise—how regularly, completely, and energetically he or she works on the assigned tasks. As already noted, the results of our research clearly indicate that the number of Take-Home Exercises fully completed by the participant was the single most powerful predictor of how much benefit the individual derived from the program as a whole. The more quickly the therapist can ascertain the origins of a group member's resistance to the program, the more quickly he or she can intervene—whether to probe the value of denial for the "ADHD skeptic" or to highlight the repeated self-denigrations of the depressed patient. Questioning the basis of failure to complete the Take-Home Exercise is, as we have suggested, important for every patient.

We present here some case examples taken from actual patients in our group treatment program, with identifying details changed to protect confidentiality. In each case, only the relevant background necessary to understand the patient's main difficulty is provided—other material from the comprehensive evaluation is not included. The patient's course of treatment in group and suggested targeted interventions in the context of the CBT program are provided for each case. We begin with a successful patient and then present profiles of an ADHD skeptic (patient in denial), an oppositional patient, a demoralized patient, and an intellectualizing obsessive patient.

THE SUCCESSFUL PATIENT

Although not yet demonstrated by empirical research, a review of our clinical observations indicates that our most successful patients appear to have some characteristics in common. They exhibit a high degree of commitment to and participation in the group—both with respect to their oral contributions in the sessions and conscientious completion of the Take-Home Exercises. They are socially responsive in that they easily become engaged in reciprocal interactions within the group with respect to supporting others and also deriving benefit from their personal accountability to the group. Successful patients may be more likely to have good social support systems outside the group as well. Successful patients are not necessarily low in comorbid anxiety or depression, but they do retain sufficient motivation and ego strength to undertake the risks of behavior change. In other words, they have reached a stage of "readiness for change" (Prochaska & Norcross, 2001). Successful patients are also more likely to be those who have no significant LDs accompanying their ADHD and thus experience fewer cognitive obstacles to implementing the strategies in daily life.

Case Study: Ron

Presenting Problems

Ron is a 38-year-old married computer salesman, who presented for the evaluation and treatment of attentional problems (e.g., drifting off in conversation), variable/inconsistent effort (e.g., difficulty seeing projects to fruition), forgetfulness (e.g., frequently forgets appointments and tasks and loses personal items), and tardiness (frequently late to work), which have collectively taken a toll on numerous aspects of his occupational functioning and personal relationships. Noted in the initial interview were restlessness and repeatedly interrupting the therapist. Ron typically drives fast (75 mph) for which he has received six speeding tickets.

Background/History

Problems surfaced early in elementary school and in many respects have persisted in breadth and intensity. Ron remembers being constantly told by teachers to "Pay attention!" and recalls comments on his report cards that indicated that he was not exercising sufficient effort and not performing to potential. He tended to do well in math and science, which came easily to him, but "hated" social science, English, and, particularly, writing composition. He was frequently chided for "clowning around" in class. Though he tended to be mischievous, he was also "charming" with teachers and avoided serious trouble. His parents, particularly his father, a math professor, were dismayed that his grades were mostly B's and C's, with a few A's, and felt he should be getting straight A's. In high school, Ron excelled at track and he feels that this "saved" him. With the support and interest of the coach, as well as his math teacher, he was able to "continue to believe in himself" and ultimately to complete high school with a 3.0 GPA.

In college, Ron immediately felt "overwhelmed." Reveling in the freedom from parental dictates and supervision, he spent more time partying than studying and began to experiment with drugs and alcohol. His grades were poor, and he was placed on academic probation at the end of the first semester. He managed to pull up his grades to a C average and, despite continued difficulties with procrastination, spotty class attendance, and incomplete or shoddy assignments, he graduated in 4 years with a major in business. After college, Ron traveled and lived abroad for a year, and upon returning, held a series of entry-level jobs in business management, typically for less than a year, before he obtained his current job in his uncle's business selling computers.

At the time of evaluation, Ron reported significant demoralization and feelings of failure (Beck score of 25). He feels self-conscious at the occasional get-togethers of his buddies from college because "they have all accomplished something with their lives and I haven't."

Beginning in his 20s, Ron has been treated intermittently for depression and anxiety, with medication (SSRIs) and psychotherapy. In addition, he and his wife of 8 years continue in marital therapy, which they entered after she threatened to leave him upon discovering that he had had an extramarital affair. She had also been disturbed by his continued overuse of alcohol and the temper outbursts that typically accompanied it. In therapy, he came to the awareness that his use of alcohol was a form of self-medication to keep painful feelings at bay, and has been able to abstain from alcohol use for the past 6 months.

Diagnoses

Ron was diagnosed with ADHD, combined type, dysthymic disorder, generalized anxiety disorder, and past alcohol dependence. He began treatment with OROS methylphenidate 6 months before group began. He reported that while on medication he was able to read the newspaper and business documents for longer periods. He also noted that he was less impulsive and less impatient—he was less inclined to speed while driving and less likely to lose his temper with his wife. However, he was still late to work and still disorganized with respect to management of time and personal belongings.

Course of Treatment in Group

During the first session, Ron shared with the group that he was extremely bored and unchallenged by his "dead-end" job. He expressed a desire to enroll in graduate school to earn an MBA, but was afraid of encountering the same difficulties he had experienced in college. He wanted to finally "get hold of the difficulties that had dogged him in [his] career and [his] marriage." Solicited for specific therapeutic goals, Ron expressed a desire to "find his focus," and more readily conquer tasks he had resisted approaching. Upon returning for the second session, Ron indicated that he had acquired a three-ring binder to organize treatment-related handouts and was able to complete the initial exercise as intended because it was relatively straightforward and not particularly challenging. Although Ron subsequently found the processes of time estimation and logging to be markedly restrictive and imposing, he also acknowledged the value/benefits associated with improved time management. Presented with the second Take-Home Exercise, calling upon him to schedule and complete a task, Ron opted to work on a client's insurance estimate; although he allocated 1½ hours to the task, unanticipated distractions (e.g., phone calls) ultimately prolonged the duration of the task. Ron nonetheless persisted and completed the task in its entirety. The group leader addressed Ron's concerns about accumulating tasks that spill over to subsequent days by encouraging him and others to consider "undercommitment" and gradually titrate up to a comfort zone of commitment.

On the heels of a successful prioritization exercise, Ron effectively connected with feelings of anxiety (e.g., related to an overdue task) that have historically contributed to and/or exacerbated tendencies to procrastinate. Ron identified the relevant automatic thought ("I've had this task since Friday and haven't started it . . . I'll never get it done"), yet acknowledged that he was unable to identify any corroborative evidence that his irrational cognition was correct. When asked to employ the positive visualization technique, Ron successfully booked a flight, hotel, rental car, and railway ticket well in advance for an upcoming vacation trip and found that having concrete cues (e.g., pictures of his travel destination) were instrumental to the success of the exercise.

Presented with specific techniques for the organization of physical space, Ron selected his home office desk, which had not been organized for many years. To help facilitate the completion of the task, Ron asked for his wife's help, and with her assistance helped to bring order to an unwieldy mess. Although he had planned to divide the surface area into sections and proceed from left to right, once he began he felt compelled to clean the area in its entirety, and created and labeled numerous file folders along the way. Following the 2½-hour exercise, Ron felt a tremendous sense of gratification and expressed confidence that the area would remain organized.

After successfully organizing a second physical space (file drawers), Ron created a plan to remove and process items from his in-box once per week to prevent them from accumulating. He proved successful at maintaining the neatness of his various zones and acknowledged that bringing various organizational tasks to fruition provided him with a sense of accomplishment.

During the final segment of the program, Ron flowcharted the components of a long-deferred plan, which was to organize his CD collection. Although he ultimately deviated somewhat from his intended plan, he felt gratified at the progress he made and brought in a photo of the collection as tangible evidence of his progress.

In a follow-up session after the end of the group program, Ron reported that he had been making steady progress. He was rarely late to work and hadn't lost his cell phone or keys in the last month. He completed an additional long-deferred project of cleaning out the garage, much to his wife's pleasure. He enrolled in an evening foreign language course at the local high school—something he had long wanted to do. Feeling generally more competent and effective, he had begun researching MBA programs, and was hoping to apply to a program in the fall.

Formulation

Despite relatively severe ADHD symptoms, long-term impairment, and a history of significant comorbidity with alcoholism, anxiety, and depression, Ron was sufficiently motivated for change at this juncture in his life that he was able to bring significant energy to bear on the process of grappling with his ADHD. As he had in high school with his teacher and coach, he was able to utilize the support of the therapist and the other group members, and to persist in his efforts even when the Take-Home Exercises proved challenging for him. The sessions concerning negative automatic thoughts helped him combat his negative self-attributions. The genuine pride and pleasure he experienced at his accomplishments helped him to maintain continued effort and solidify his gains.

THE ADHD SKEPTIC (THE PATIENT IN DENIAL)

The ADHD skeptic has not fully accepted that he or she has ADHD—or, perhaps, that it even exists! Propensities toward depression may contribute to the maintenance of denial in order to protect vulnerable self-esteem. Some patients enroll in group treatment despite their ambivalence about the diagnosis. In many cases, the identification with and support of other group members, combined with psychoeducation about ADHD, helps them to get past their denial and to begin to cope actively with their difficulties. Other patients, like the one profiled below, do not make that transition within the first treatment program, and may have to initiate a return at a later date when they have greater readiness for change.

Case Study: Regina

Presenting Problems

Regina is a 28-year-old unmarried graduate art student, who presented to the program with concerns regarding restlessness (e.g., inability to work on an art project on the computer without getting up 15–25 times a day), distractibility (e.g., struggles to maintain focus while reading), and difficulties with time management (e.g., requires the threat of unpalatable consequences to compel her to undertake a task). Also noted were vacillations between intervals of extreme organization and disorganization, and repeated misplacement of possessions.

In addition to these concerns, Regina characterized herself as impulsive and judgmental, and conceded that there were situations in which she divulged information too rapidly, and in ways that might be construed as offensive. Finally, Regina acknowledged being digressive during conversations, a pattern that was observed during the clinical interview as well.

Contributing to Regina's variable personal and professional engagement were reports of being "either very depressed or in a zone." She experienced prior but not current depressive episodes, including suicidal ideation. She depicted herself as "eccentric, the odd person out; on the outside looking in."

Background/History

Regina was initially diagnosed with ADHD during childhood; however, her mother, who was a registered nurse, adamantly opposed psychopharmacological treatment, and over the years provided Regina with literature questioning the legitimacy of the disorder and highlighting possible repercussions of pharmacological treatment.

At age 23, Regina pursued individual counseling with a clinical social worker following a breakup with her boyfriend; however, treatment was reportedly discontinued after four to five sessions. Most recently, Regina pursued psychopharmacological treatment of depression for 4 months prior to the evaluation. She also received trials of Strattera and Wellbutrin, both of which precipitated negative side effects and were not deemed therapeutically beneficial. At the time of the current assessment, Regina was receiving treatment with a very small dose of Ritalin (5 mg as needed). The medication reportedly helped her to "consume more information," but allegedly triggered heart palpitations and angina.

Diagnoses

As a result of this evaluation, Regina was diagnosed with the following: ADHD, combined type; major depressive disorder in partial remission; and anxiety disorder not otherwise specified (current).

Course of Treatment in Group

At the first group session, Regina acknowledged feeling skeptical regarding the diagnostic validity of ADHD, suggesting that her problems were experienced to some degree by everyone and, in her own case, were largely restricted to tasks that were mundane and/ or less intrinsically rewarding. Her skepticism notwithstanding, Regina remained open to a supportive experience in group and to the possibility of acquiring strategies to address difficulties in the realms of time management, organization, and planning. In group she was otherwise personable and displayed an engaging sense of humor.

Upon returning for the second session, Regina indicated that she completed the Take-Home Exercise a day earlier than she intended, and dismissed it as "not a big deal." She continued to harbor skepticism about ADHD, however, citing her ability to complete tasks when provided with rigid timetables or deadlines. Regina scheduled but did not execute the initial task for her second Take-Home Exercise and rebuffed the notion that contingent self-reinforcement might facilitate its completion. She viewed the need for rewards as juvenile and suggested that she, like many others, would be able to complete the task right before it was due. At this point, the therapist encouraged her to envision the pitfalls of deferring the activity until immediately before the expected completion date (e.g., unforeseen distractions or expectations arise, inaccurate estimation of what might be involved in completing a task, stress of completing the task under pressure). As the group progressed, Regina reiterated yet simultaneously downplayed the significance of her inability to initiate certain activities in the absence of concrete deadlines. Later in the program, while exploring the factors that might contribute to her inertia, Regina indicated that certain automatic thoughts (e.g., "should" statements, all-or-none thinking) tended to be her most formidable obstacles to task initiation.

In contrast to her approach to time-management exercises, Regina was generally more successful at creation and maintenance of organizational structures. Prior to the tenth session, Regina contacted the group leader to indicate that professional obligations/ responsibilities would hamper continued participation and did not attend any further sessions.

Formulation

Regina's reluctance to come to terms with the legitimacy of the diagnosis appeared to constrain her engagement in the group process (e.g., she tended not to provide constructive comments or feedback to fellow members). Although Regina at times put forth adequate effort to complete the Take-Home Exercises, she frequently dismissed her accomplishments and generally characterized her experiences in a disaffected, somewhat listless manner. Importantly, Regina's identification with several of the cognitive distortions highlights the role of emotional factors in her procrastination/task avoidance. Although her failure to complete the group program may speak to difficulties managing time and following through on commitments, it also appears likely that Regina never fully came to terms with her diagnostic status and, therefore, did not prioritize the program's therapeutic interventions accordingly.

Suggested Therapeutic Interventions

For clients such as Regina, targeted efforts early in the program to confront skeptical beliefs and attitudes may heighten preparedness for change. In particular, such individuals may be queried early during the program regarding the relative value of maintaining versus surrendering their resistance. For other clients, this process may have to go on during a period of individual psychotherapy before they are ready to undertake the group treatment, as described further in Chapter 5.

THE OPPOSITIONAL PATIENT

The oppositional patient is resistant either to the notion that he or she has ADHD or to the possibility that he or she can change or improve. The oppositional patient has features of the ADHD skeptic, but has built a stronger bulwark of defenses. Patients who continue to question the diagnosis often harbor the belief that they *should* be able to complete tasks, focus, maintain organization, and so forth. This belief is typically rooted in childhood experiences with parents who may have been overly moralistic or judgmental and who failed to recognize that the patient's difficulties in childhood were manifestations of a condition over which the child lacked full control. The persistence of this belief into adulthood allows the patient to continue to believe in his or her essential complete self-control and potential perfectibility. The belief often masks underlying feelings of incompetence and fears of failure should he or she attempt to change and not succeed. Early in the program oppositional patients may begin to denigrate the therapy and/or the therapist's competence, typically expounding on why they are convinced the program will not work for them. Avoiding completion of the Take-Home Exercise simultaneously allows the patient to avoid the possibility of yet another failure experience and confirms his or her a priori belief that therapy does not work. Oppositional patients may also be attempting to "hold on" to their ADHD symptoms as a defense against having to confront more serious personality issues, as the following case illustrates.

Case Study: Craig

Presenting Problems

Craig is a 40-year-old married engineer who states that his "personal life is a mess" and presents now with problems of disorganization. He is "overwhelmed" with everyday tasks including mundane tasks at home, tracking his finances, and completing reports and other paperwork at his job.

Background/History

Craig's problems with task completion and organization had an onset in third grade when he particularly remembers having difficulty with essay writing and with memorization. These problems continued through high school. In his first year in college, he remembers feeling "overwhelmed" by the amount of reading necessary. Throughout college he experienced great anxiety while preparing for tests, for which he took an antianxiety medication for 2–3 weeks at the end of each semester. Because of failure to complete term projects in a timely fashion, he took numerous "incompletes," which delayed his graduation by a year and a half.

Diagnosis

As a result of the evaluation, Craig was diagnosed with ADHD, inattentive type.

Course of Treatment in Group

From the outset, Craig openly and frequently challenged the therapist by stating or implying that the program would not be effective for him. For example, he resisted doing a task proposed for the Take-Home Exercise with the comment that, as a person with ADHD, he would *never* be able to complete tasks efficiently. He thereupon amplified the reasons why a person with ADHD would have difficulty doing the task, implying that we, as therapists, either didn't understand the nature of ADHD or were ineffective. He recited the different approaches he had tried that had proved ineffective for him over the previous decades. His stance was "Since nothing has worked for me in the past, nothing ever will."

In a subsequent session, Craig shared his difficulties completing household tasks like repairs and bill paying, which he found to be particularly difficult and anxiety arousing, causing him to procrastinate until the bills were overdue. He noted that such tasks took many times longer than they should because he was stymied by not having the necessary materials. He found these obstacles frustrating and lost his momentum as he forgot or otherwise failed to complete the intermediate steps. He acknowledged that when he was finally able to complete a task, he was reinforced by a feeling of relief. However, he believed that if he did complete the task on a timely basis he would just feel "aimless or adrift" and wonder what he should do next. He would not be inclined to actively reward himself, but instead would more likely tell himself that he "should have been able to do it anyway." The therapist highlighted that this difficulty reinforcing oneself and tendency to self-berate undermined progress and caused persistent demoralization.

By the midpoint of the program, Craig continued to articulate the view that the Take-Home Exercises were "pointless"—that, for example, he would never be able to commit to using one planner because, as a person with ADHD, he would always need to seek out stimulation and change, which would include having to continually change to new planner systems. He appeared to adhere to this view even as the therapist and the group members highlighted the negativistic and self-defeating thinking implicit in his statements. He made a partially successful attempt to complete the Take-Home Exercise that involved listing, prioritizing, and scheduling weekend to-do items in the planner. At the next session, he reported that he succeeded only in making lists of the tasks to be accomplished and acknowledged to the group that he felt "overwhelmed and confused" when he tried to schedule them. He was given support and reinforcement for making partial progress. After the seventh session, Craig appeared to give up trying to complete the Take-Home Exercises altogether, complaining that they were "overwhelming" and "time-consuming" for him. From this point onward, he also arrived late to the sessions, participated less, and frequently was observed to have his head down, writing something irrelevant or doodling. In one of these sessions, he confided to the group more about his difficulties in prioritizing and decision making. He believed that he delayed making decisions because after he did so, he would be at loose ends, wondering what to do next. These comments suggested, as did his previous comments concerning reluctance to self-reinforce, that he experienced underlying depression and a sense of self as being inadequate, which he warded off by perpetuating disorganized, frenetic activity. His strong resistance to taking any steps toward making change or trying new strategies suggests that Craig has a strong subconscious investment in maintaining his symptoms. At the end of the program, Craig despaired of ever being able to make any headway since he "had tried so many times unsuccessfully in the past."

Formulation

Craig's difficulties completing the Take-Home Exercises and his articulation of expectations for failure were early clues to his powerful resistance to change. His fragile ego was so easily wounded when he was unable to live up to his own or others' expectations that it was much less painful to debunk these expectations at the outset. These problems were addressed in the group by highlighting the self-defeating and demoralizing nature of his expectations and predictions. Whereas interventions of this type, articulated by both the therapist and other group members, are often helpful in overcoming participants' fears of failure and resistance to change, in Craig's case they were insufficient. An additional challenge for the therapist in this case was Craig's need to share the blame for his difficulties with others (including the therapist) who were expecting him to accomplish these "impossible" tasks and, indeed, were ultimately attempting to break through his self-protective defenses.

Although Craig apparently made little progress toward assimilating better self-management skills, he did seem to get in touch with some of the underlying feelings of depression that his persistent disorganization had served to mask. He was aware, on some level, that if he did get a grip on these difficulties, he would have to confront his inner sense of emptiness and inadequacy. It became clear that these issues would have to be addressed in individual psychotherapy before Craig would be able to make any real progress in coping with the cognitive and behavioral manifestations of his ADHD.

Patients like Craig typically arouse frustrated, angry feelings on the part of therapists because their comments may be felt to be offensive—implying that the therapist is not competent, for example—and because they are help-rejecting, parrying away the therapist's best efforts. It can be quite difficult to continue to be patient and supportive with this kind of patient.

Suggested Therapeutic Interventions

In the group setting, the therapist can first elicit reasons for the patient's failure to complete homework, which, for oppositional/resistant patients, will likely elicit beliefs that it "won't work." As appropriate in the course of the group, the therapist can highlight the cognitive distortions (e.g., "fortune-teller error") that underlie this belief, with statements like the following:

> "You seem to be saying that because nothing has worked for you in the past, nothing ever will."
> "You seem to be saying that 'because this is how I've been, this is how I always will be.'"
> "You seem to be assuming that this won't work without having actually tried it."

As the patient becomes more comfortable with greater intimacy in the group setting, the therapist may have opportunities to begin to uncover the patient's fear of change—to identify what he or she is guarding against—by posing an open-ended question such as "I wonder how your life would be different if you didn't have these problems." It is likely, however, that these difficulties will have to be addressed in individual psychotherapy.

THE DEMORALIZED PATIENT

The demoralized or depressed patient is "stuck." He or she complains of having made little progress toward personal goals and despairs of ever being able to do so. He or she tends to be irritable and frustrated with him- or herself. Accomplishments are downplayed and feelings of inadequacy and self-criticism are frequently voiced. The depressed or demoralized patient may appear to be superficially compliant with the treatment program. As in the case described below, he or she may appear to dutifully carry out the Take-Home Exercises, but in so doing, chooses easily acquitted tasks that lend a feeling of accomplishment while avoiding tackling the issues, problems, or tasks that are of major importance but ego threatening.

Case Study: Laura

Presenting Problems

Laura is a 40-year-old never-married freelance journalist. She presents with concerns related to difficulty with focused attention, "management of time and paper," planning, and organization. Since obtaining her master's degree in journalism at the age of 30, she has held one full-time job with a newspaper, but has had no permanent employment in the last 3 years. Her freelance income is insufficient to her needs. The disorganization and clutter in her home makes her reluctant to socialize at home. Her social life suffers more generally due to inefficiency that leaves little time to cultivate meaningful relationships. She often feels lonely, worries about her future, and is chronically frustrated by the lack of progress in her life.

Background/History

Laura grew up with her biological parents as an only child. Her father is an accomplished lawyer and her mother a full-time homemaker. Her parents were often critical of her efforts unless she was at the top of her class. She attended competitive private schools where her performance was generally average or above. As early as second grade she had difficulty listening in class and a propensity to wander around the classroom, blurt out answers, and talk too much. She also fatigued easily when learning new information, lost things, and made frequent careless mistakes. School records obtained from her parents underscored such difficulties in childhood.

In college and journalism school, Laura had difficulty listening in lectures and taking clear notes. She compensated by taping every lecture. She was later dismissed from two journalism positions with newspapers because she failed to meet deadlines and because her submissions were often poorly edited. Although she has made intermittent efforts to find a permanent position in her field, her lack of success has made her feel increasingly despondent about her abilities and long-term prospects.

Diagnoses

The evaluation concluded that Laura had ADHD, combined type; and dysthymia. Despite recommendations to pursue a pharmacological consultation to treat ADHD and depression, Laura declined, saying she was opposed to medication generally.

Course of Treatment

At the first session Laura appeared physically tired and expressed that she felt "stagnant" in her life and her career. She complained of being exactly where she was 3 years ago, which, in her case, was still unemployed. The group was appropriately empathic with her concerns and attempted to encourage her to be hopeful and to pursue alternative networking avenues. The goals she identified for herself in the program were to create organization in her home, decrease clutter, and dismantle complex tasks, such as searching for a job, into more manageable chunks.

During the first quarter of the group program, Laura repeatedly described being frustrated and irritated by her lack of success. She complained that she had items on her to-do list that had been there for months and that transferring these items to subsequent days had little utility other than to remind her of the little she accomplished, causing her to feel badly about herself. Further probing revealed that Laura underestimated how long tasks took to complete, and expected to accomplish too much daily. When experiencing disappointment she worked more slowly and spent most of her time tied to tasks that were easy. Tasks such as responding to e-mail provided her immediate rewards (e.g., a sense of completion) but consumed much of her time, leaving little time for the long-term planning and follow-through required of her job search.

The Take-Home Exercise to complete an automatic thought log elicited thoughts such as "I'm so dumb" and "I can't understand anything." Laura also noted that when she doesn't receive a response to an e-mail she assumed that she had irritated the other party or that she was not worthy of his or her time and attention. She agreed that her thinking might be distorted and identified distortions such as "disqualifying the positive" and "mind reading." However, the quickness with which she provided counterarguments to challenge these thoughts appeared superficial; she maintained a slight smile and her affect remained composed throughout. She argued that her track record indicated that her negative self-assessment was valid, and then simply smiled and nodded when others challenged these beliefs. She continued to minimize her accomplishments by simultaneously highlighting her perceived inadequacies, such as working slowly and lack of self-discipline.

During the second half of the program, Laura made some gains in organizing her home office. She identified three zones, which she worked at organizing systematically. Her job search, however, presented the most obstacles and discussion brought to light considerable anxiety about the likelihood of her being able to function as a full-time journalist should she obtain such a job. The final planning project was employed to assist her in breaking down her job search. This included exploration of the areas of journalism where she could be most effective, and the feelings she had about continuing her pursuit. She was highly ambivalent about taking on this project, which she described as "emotionally charged." By the end of the program Laura had made little progress on the final project. She avoided the tasks and complained that her current contract work left her with little time and energy to tackle them.

Formulation

Although Laura acknowledged her diagnosis of ADHD and depression in the abstract, she was unable to utilize the group to experience negative emotions and mourn the loss of an ideal self, generated, in part, by unrealistic and unfulfilled parental expectations of her performance and behavior in childhood. She was drawn to tasks that were easily accomplished and allowed her to maintain her perfectionism and her self-reliance. This may also help to explain her rejection of pharmacotherapy. Within the group format, she was able to acknowledge her feelings and fears of inadequacy, but was reluctant to become vulnerable to sadness. Moreover, it was difficult for her and for the others in the group to adequately tease out her realistic perceptions from her cognitive distortions.

Patients such as Laura may initially trigger feelings of frustration and irritation in the therapist at the lack of progress. Therapists and group members may be drawn to quick strategies to address the difficulties with practical goals (e.g., job search), rather than identifying the perceived hopelessness and depression. As the patient becomes more attuned to his or her feelings, the therapist may empathize with the feelings of sadness and anxiety related to lost time and opportunities, and to acceptance of the self as imperfect.

Suggested Therapeutic Interventions

It is likely that patients like Laura will require individual therapy to fully explore and address intermingled depression and ADHD, and, in particular, to tease out cognitive distortions from accurate perceptions. Within the group context, it is important to encourage such patients to select tasks for the Take-Home Exercises that relate to areas of deficit and meaningful short- and long-term goals, while simultaneously reinforcing positive effort and helping them to identify and revise unrealistic expectations. To the extent comfortably possible in group, one might also encourage self-disclosure, and identify and gently challenge avoidant behavior when it occurs.

THE INTELLECTUALIZING OBSESSIONAL PATIENT

The intellectualizing patient can at first seem like the ideal patient, devoted as he or she apparently is to thinking in psychological terms, actively processing observations and making interpretations. This type of patient can seduce the therapist into believing that he or she is highly successful in communicating with and leading him or her to new insights. Over time, however, it becomes apparent that the patient's extensive self-analysis is actually an intellectualizing defense that simultaneously protects against change and masks the resistance to it.

Case Study: Max

Presenting Problems

Max is a self-referred 37-year-old single second-year law student who complained of difficulty completing written assignments in a timely manner. He attributed these delays to problems with time estimation and organization of ideas. He reported similar problems in his personal life including failure to complete bill paying and other household management tasks, poor time management, poor planning, and poor management of personal belongings. Concurrently, Max reported perfectionism and test anxiety, and had received insight-oriented therapy for treatment of depression in the past.

Background/History

Max reported lifelong difficulties with focused attention and task completion. The only son of two professionals, he was a very smart, precocious, and hyperactive child who recalled no overt academic struggles throughout most of his schooling until his senior year in high school. At that time he experienced difficulty completing his senior thesis "every step of the way." He nonetheless graduated with honors and gained entry to an Ivy League university. He reveled in the freedom he found on campus and immediately became involved with several on-campus political and activist groups, which often took precedence over his academic work. He frequently missed classes, and was late with assignments and term papers, completing them after "all-nighters" or taking incompletes in the courses. He changed his major subject several times to correspond with his evolving interests in politics, philosophy, and Eastern religions. He was able to complete college within 4 years with a few A's but otherwise generally poor to mediocre grades—much less than he felt he could have achieved had he applied himself more diligently. Having no plan for a career or graduate work after college, Max worked for several nonprofit social justice and environmental groups and later did freelance writing while he traveled through Europe and Asia. In his mid-30s he enrolled in law school but quickly experienced a recurrence of the academic organizational difficulties he experienced in college. At the time of his participation in the group he was on academic probation.

The family history is positive for mood, anxiety, and learning disorders.

Diagnoses

Max was diagnosed with the following: ADHD, combined type; anxiety disorder not otherwise specified; and depressive disorder not otherwise specified, in remission. At the time of the evaluation and enrollment in group, he was taking bupropion, an SSRI, and mixed amphetamine salts (Adderall).

Course of Treatment in Group

Max initially overtly appeared very compliant and cooperative. He attended all sessions, generally arrived on time, and spoke frequently about the implications of all new material and how it applied to his life. He readily volunteered to discuss and explore his own struggles and empathized with those of others. Max appeared to be very insightful. He made intelligent comments, discussing with ease and appropriately applying the concepts, principles, and techniques of the sessions. For example, when the group leader once left the room to make phone calls while group members filled out forms, he laughingly commented about the leader taking advantage of a "time crack." On other occasions, he thoughtfully shared insights about others' automatic thoughts and possible underlying cognitive distortions, as well as possible ways to dispute them.

During the course of the sessions, however, it became apparent that Max was completing the Take-Home Exercises only partially at best. During the reviews of the exercises, he was quite voluble in analyzing and explaining why he behaved in the way he did, both in general and with respect to the exercises. He shared concerns about compatibility between his own temperament and personality style and the scripted exercises. He questioned, in existential fashion, whether he truly *wanted* to complete the task, organize the space, and so on. He continued to manifest resistance to changing the way he organized his day, and described the measurement of time as an "external dimension that [he] was rebelling against."

Given consistent therapist and group feedback, by the midpoint of the program Max had become increasingly aware that he frequently expended more energy in resisting and rationalizing his resistance, than in carrying out the task itself, and he began to work harder to complete the exercises. He sought to understand why he was "very good at completing 99% of everything" but "unable to finish anything." He applied the cognitive-behavioral principles discussed in the group, and identified the "critical committee in [his] head" that oversaw and evaluated his work, leading both to performance anxiety and to an adversarial attitude toward teachers and bosses. He also voiced the interesting observation that he was not able to be organized, because he was "not deserving of the success" that organization connotes.

Formulation

Max's frequent, lengthy, and apparently insightful comments and observations at first served to mask how little he was actually *doing* outside the group sessions. His failures to complete the Take-Home Exercises were well rationalized during the early reviews of the exercises and suggested to the therapist that he was indeed doing his best to cooperate with the program. As his resistance to implementing *any* of the suggested strategies became more apparent, however, the defensive nature of his intellectualization became more apparent as well. Max came to be more aware in the sessions that he was reluctant to give up his ADHD symptoms because they provided a ready "excuse" if he ultimately was not as successful as he expected of himself or others expected of him. Fearing negative evaluation, rejection, or criticism, completing only 99% of a task allowed him to retain the illusion of control over what he actually produced and also served to delay the moment of final reckoning. Also, as he noted, completing one task simply meant that another was on its way.

Max's interesting and articulate self-analysis served as a "smoke screen" to ward off more penetrating awareness by himself or others. His intellectualizing defenses protected him from receiving criticism, or disappointing himself or others. Simultaneously, they engaged the therapist in a way that allowed him or her to preserve an illusion of his or her efficacy in rendering the treatment.

Suggested Therapeutic Interventions

This case illustrates both the importance of carefully tracking completion of the Take-Home Exercises, and the therapist's dilemma of discerning the appropriate degree of pressure to exert on a participant without causing embarrassment in the group situation. Early in the group program, the therapist may consider gently confronting and exploring the patient's pattern of verbal acquiescence coupled with behavioral noncompliance. As the group progresses, and more personal history is shared, the therapist might validate the patient's history of chronically "disappointing" others and generalize this issue for discussion in the group. Throughout, as with all patients, it would be particularly important to support and reinforce the patient in his or her attempts to complete the Take-Home Exercises.

SUMMARY

The foregoing cases illustrate how individual differences in comorbidity, personality, and/or defensive style may be recognized and addressed within the group context. In some cases, patients like the foregoing may benefit from a course of individual therapy concurrent with or after a course of group treatment. Adaptation of group CBT for individual treatment is described in the next chapter.

CHAPTER 5

Modifying the Treatment for Use in Individual Therapy

JEANETTE WASSERSTEIN, MARY V. SOLANTO, *and* DAVID J. MARKS

The CBT approach is easily adapted for use in individual therapy. This allows the therapist to personalize the treatment for individual needs with respect to specific skills deficits, business or personal circumstances, tasks and responsibilities, pace of treatment, and emotional obstacles to change. In addition, patients with certain comorbidities, for whom the group modality is not appropriate, may benefit from individual therapy.

WHEN INDIVIDUAL THERAPY IS THE BETTER OPTION

Individual therapy allows for tailoring the treatment to individual needs. Although most adults with ADHD have difficulty in both time management and physical organization, there are some who have little difficulty in organization and thus can benefit from an exclusive focus on efficient use of time. (Few to none have no difficulty in time management.) The individual modality also allows for adaptation of the strategies to the particular demands and work environments typical of different occupations and professions. The writer, for example, has to be able to organize ideas on paper and to work without distraction on one project for significant blocks of time. The lawyer, on the other hand, may have to track the progress of multiple cases, responding in a timely fashion to the changing demands of each. Strategies to facilitate sustained attention and resistance to distraction may have prominent importance for the writer, whereas task initiation, track-

65

ing, attentional shifting, and aids to support working memory may be more important for the lawyer.

A second advantage is that the pace of treatment may be tailored to the individual. Some patients may be able to progress more quickly than the group's timetable allows. Others, particularly those with learning impairments, may need more time to work through, rehearse, and ultimately assimilate some or all of the strategies. In some of these cases, an appropriate alternative may be individual sessions *concurrent* with the group program to allow for more intensive support, elaboration, and rehearsal.

Third, many patients with ADHD experience strong emotional resistance to change. Although these issues are addressed in the group program, some individuals, like those described in the last chapter, who are in denial of their ADHD, or who are highly oppositional, depressed, demoralized, perfectionistic, or fearful of failure may need a period of individual treatment during which these issues can be addressed.

Finally, circumstances may render individual treatment more feasible for some individuals, including those who wish to minimize the risk of public exposure to the community, and those who cannot coordinate group treatment meetings with their schedules.

WHEN GROUP TREATMENT IS INADVISABLE

Among those who need intervention to develop cognitive self-management skills but for whom the group format is a less appropriate modality, are individuals with a spectrum of problematic comorbid conditions, and/or those with more unique treatment needs. This subset of patients includes (1) those who could disrupt the group process—for example, clients with aggressive tendencies who would alienate other group members; (2) those with severe social phobia who may be extremely uncomfortable in social settings; and (3) patients with other more severe forms of psychopathology, which either cannot be appropriately addressed or managed in the group setting, or alternatively, reflect another critical clinical matter requiring more immediate attention. This latter cluster includes people with borderline personality disorder, suicidal ideation or intent, and individuals with active substance abuse or dependency.

ASSESSMENT AND PLANNING FOR INDIVIDUAL THERAPY

Most people with ADHD have a mixture of executive function deficits that do not cluster in predictable patterns. For example, some cannot prioritize or initiate, others cannot estimate time, others cannot track or organize space, and so on. Thus, in order to be optimally effective, the therapist must evaluate the landscape of the individual's deficits and strengths. Since the program is highly structured, sessions may be selected from the group program according to the needs of the patient in individual treatment. Sessions 2–6 in the group program address time management, Sessions 7–9 deal with organization, and Sessions 10–12 deal with planning (see table of contents of the Treatment Manual on p. 87).

The Guided Inquiry of Skills Form at the end of this chapter provides a guide for the therapist to conduct a systematic inquiry into the individual's executive functions and self-management skills. To facilitate an understanding of context, the interview begins with an inquiry into the individual's duties and responsibilities at home and at work, as well as his or her long- and short-term goals, personal reinforcers, and negative contingencies. The body of Form 5.1 guides the therapist to systematically inquire about vulnerable skills (e.g., estimating time, setting up a filing system) and executive functions (e.g., initiation, inhibition, sustained attention, planning), as well as task-specific areas of potential difficulty (e.g., sorting the mail, paying bills). The contribution of emotional problems (e.g., demoralization, perfectionism) is noted. However, much more information concerning these will presumably be derived from the comprehensive diagnostic evaluation that precedes the treatment.

The corresponding Hierarchy of Skills Keyed to Sessions (Table 5.1) indicates, in the middle column, the strategies or skills necessary to address each dysfunction or deficit identified in the left-hand column and, in the right-hand column, the session number(s) in which they may be found. Each session has a Take-Home Exercise that can be assigned, repeated, expanded, or modified. For example, a patient with particular difficulty with time awareness might complete multiple time-estimation or time-logging exercises, while spending little time on organizing zones, initiation exercises, or disputing automatic thoughts. Another may need to focus on setting priorities and scheduling both short (daily or weekly planner) and long term (more complex projects). Yet another may need to focus on negative attributions and how these are immobilizing, opening the road to more conventional psychotherapeutic interventions coupled with targeted skill building. Ultimately, the individualized approach can be more flexible and targeted, while remaining programmatic.

It is also useful for the therapist and the patient to have a *metaview* of the executive function supports or skills the program teaches. Through this type of understanding the therapist can better identify where the patient needs the most intervention. Categories include:

• **Self-management techniques:** dismantling tasks into smaller components, contingent self-reinforcement, visualization of rewards/consequences, recognizing and disputing automatic thoughts, establishing repetitive rhythms of behaviors (e.g., regular day for grocery shopping or laundry), and environmental manipulations (e.g., decrease distractors, increase structure, make appointments with self in a paper or computerized planner)

TABLE 5.1. Hierarchy of Skills Keyed to Sessions

Hierarchy of skills	Strategy	Session
1. Wears a watch daily.	• Discuss benefits	2
2. Planner.	• Methods and benefits of planner use • Prioritizing	2 4
3. Gets to bed and awakens at the desired time.	• Proper evening and next-day planning • Use of alarms and incentives • Stops/inhibits current activity	4, optional
4. Gets to work, appointments, and other engagements on time.	• Time estimation and planning • Stops/inhibits current activity	2

5. Daily task completion
  a. Has a plan for the day.
  b. Has a plan for the week.
	• Review use of task lists to prioritize and plan a schedule for the day and week	4

c. Initiates tasks on time.	• Proper time estimation • Break down tasks into manageable chunks • Contingent self-reward • Overcome anxious avoidance	2 3 5
d. Avoids or overcomes distractions.	• Set up workplace to avoid physical and human distractions	7, 8
e. Completes tasks on time.	• Proper time estimation • Break down tasks into manageable chunks • Contingent self-reward	2 3 3
f. Stops (inhibits) tasks appropriately.	• Self-notification (alarm) • Avoid overfocusing	
6. Long-term projects a. Planning	• Use of flowchart	10
b. Completion	• Visualization of long-term rewards	6
7. Organization	• Setting up, implementing, and maintaining organizational systems	7, 8, 9
8. Emotional issues	• Identify and address "automatic thoughts" during inquiry of Take-Home Exercise and throughout session as appropriate • Repeat thought log as needed	5

- **Time-management skills:** creating task lists, time estimation, prioritization, flow-charting, and scheduling in a paper or computerized planner.

- **Space-management techniques:** creating zones for related possessions (everything has a "home"), user-friendly positioning of materials (e.g., keys by the entry), "File–Action–Trash" (FAT) system for sorting all accumulated materials (clothing, books, papers, etc.).

IMPLEMENTING INDIVIDUAL THERAPY

Setting and Adhering to the Agenda

Behavioral and cognitive-behavioral therapies in general and CBT for ADHD in particular, require that the therapist adhere to a specific agenda and procedures in order to achieve the goals of treatment. Whereas the group format lends itself to structured presentation and discussion, it is easy for the therapist in individual CBT to be drawn into discussion of the patient's day-to-day issues, crises, and problems. The therapist may quickly find him- or herself "putting out fires" rather than working systematically to remediate deficits and enhance skills. This risk may be minimized by presenting at the outset of treatment an overview of the program and its methods, and describing the usual format of each session.

At each session, the therapist must strive to maintain a balance between adhering to the agenda, on the one hand, and maintaining rapport with the patient and dealing with emotional crises, on the other. Toward that end, at the start of each session, the therapist listens to the patient's presenting comments and concerns. If these are not relevant to the Take-Home Exercise or the strategies under discussion, the therapist must judge whether the material represents a valid emotional concern, or a logistical obstacle subserving resistance. The therapist must further determine whether the issue is sufficiently prepotent that it must be addressed immediately or whether it can be deferred to the later part of the session. If the latter, the therapist may say something like "It sounds like this [issue] is concerning and upsetting to you. But we also want to make sure that we stay focused and on track so let us devote [specified] minutes to discussing the Take-Home Exercise of last week, and then devote the remaining time to the discussion of [current issue]." It may be the case that the issue is sufficiently complex (e.g., significant problems in a primary relationship, preparing graduate school applications, career or job choice) that it requires exclusive focus in one or more sessions, in which case a plan can be made to designate future sessions for that purpose. Not coincidentally, the therapist is here modeling good time management (including time estimation, prioritizing, planning, and scheduling), which can be explicitly called to the patient's attention.

Another pitfall in individual treatment is the temptation to bypass presentation of the material provided to group members at each session. It may feel too "formal" to present didactic material to a patient in a one-to-one session—particularly for therapists for whom dialogue constitutes the prime modus operandi of treatment. This background material, however, is important in that it elucidates the specific deficits in ADHD and provides a detailed rationale for the strategies presented in that session, thereby facilitating their assimilation and generalization to the patient's everyday life.

A reasonable allocation of time in the individual session would be 10–15 minutes for review of the Take-Home Exercise, 20 minutes for introduction and discussion of new material, and 10–15 minutes for explanation of and anticipatory troubleshooting of the next Take-Home Exercise.

Review of the Take-Home Exercise

An important advantage of individual therapy over group therapy is that it allows for more in-depth review of the patient's experience with the Take-Home Exercise, particularly with respect to addressing emotional or logistical issues that may be interfering with completion. As in the group program, each individual therapy session begins with a review of the Take-Home Exercise, including an inquiry concerning reasons for non- or partial completion. The therapist and patient together analyze the process and outcome of the exercise, with a goal of exploring reasons for success and for difficulty, and identifying other strategies that might have been utilized effectively instead or in addition.

The therapist should inquire about the Take-Home Exercise in a sensitive and supportive manner. It is important to help patients understand at the outset that it is expected that some of the exercises will be challenging, but that working through these difficulties provides "grist for the mill" of treatment that is ultimately effective. It is important as well to reinforce the patient for effort and for successive approximations to a fully successful result.

It is also critical that the individual therapist query the causes of failures to attempt the exercise or halfhearted superficial efforts. Although there of course may be extenuating circumstances that prevent completion of the exercise (illness, unanticipated conflicting obligations, or other crises), repeated excuses or superficial efforts may signal the presence of depression or demoralization, anxiety or fear of failure, or oppositionality or denial of the diagnosis. Indeed, resistance shows up most rapidly in the patient's approach to the Take-Home Exercise. It is important for the therapist to listen with the proverbial "third ear" since deep-seated conflicts can also contribute to poor compliance. For example, success inhibition and/or issues around a history of abuse can complicate and exacerbate ordinary ADHD symptoms (see Bemporad, 2001, for discussion). The individual therapy provides a setting wherein these emotional obstacles can be identified and addressed in a timely fashion in comfort and privacy. It is well to bear in mind that efficacy studies of cognitive-behavioral interventions, including our own (see Chapter 6), have repeatedly shown that completion of the Take-Home Exercise is a critical component of treatment that is significantly related to positive outcomes.

Finally, as in group therapy, it is important to remind the patient that it is expected that he or she will *continue* to utilize the strategies introduced in each new Take-Home Exercise, such that they become part of the individual's daily self-management repertoire.

Termination

Planning for termination can begin when (1) the patient appears to have mastered the CBT strategies and incorporated them into everyday life or (2) when the focus of treatment has shifted to emotional issues (such as anxiety, depression, PTSD, or personality disorders) and the therapist believes his or her skills are no longer aligned with the needs of the patient.

Readministration of standardized measures like the CAARS, the On Time Management, Organization, and Planning Scale (ON-TOP), or the BRIEF can be helpful in ascertaining the extent of improvement and identifying any areas of residual concern. If time and resources permit, it is sensible to allow for a period of extended "maintenance" treatment after treatment proper has concluded, during which the therapist and patient can observe how well the benefits are maintained during the stressors of daily life, and/ or reinforce continued practice of the skills during the inevitably changing situational demands. A reasonable maintenance sequence might be prescheduled sessions, at a frequency of about once per month, for the first 3–6 months, followed by additional sessions on an as-needed basis.

In other respects, the usual termination principles and processes apply to termination of CBT. That is, the therapist reviews with the patient the progress that has been made in the course of treatment—specifically identifying the new strategies learned, habits changed, and insights attained—and anticipates with the patient what difficulties might arise in the future and how these might be recognized and addressed. It may also be very useful to summarize the relevant strategies in written form as a tool for future reference. The Take-Home Notes for Session 12 may serve this purpose well. Patients should also be made aware of community resources to which they may turn for support and information, including Children and Adults with Attention Deficit/Hyperactivity Disorder (CHADD) and the Attention Deficit Disorder Association (ADDA), on the national level and any local groups that may be available. In addition, it is very reassuring to patients to know that "the door is always open" (if, of course, this is true), should they wish to return to refresh their skills, or obtain help with new difficulties. Indeed, given that ADHD is a chronic condition, it is not at all unusual for patients to come back to treatment after a period away in order to renew or expand their skills.

FORM 5.1. Guided Inquiry of Skills

Name: _____ Date: _____ Therapist: _____

To the therapist: Conduct an inquiry of the following:

Major Tasks/Duties/Responsibilities:

At home:

_____

_____

_____

At work:

_____

_____

_____

Personal Goals and Priorities:

Short term:

_____

_____

Long term:

_____

_____

Personal Rewards:

_____

_____

_____

Personal Contingencies (i.e., anticipated rewards or consequences contingent on effort or output): _____

_____

_____

Continue on reverse if necessary.

(cont.)

Hierarchy of Skills	Yes	No	Comments
1. Wears a watch daily.			
2. Planner			
a. Has an appropriate planner.			
b. Schedules all appointments in planner.			
c. Maintains to-do (task) lists in planner.			
d. Prioritizes and schedules tasks in planner.			
e. Checks planner regularly.			
3. Gets to bed and awakens at the desired time.			
4. Gets to work, appointments, and other engagements on time.			
5. Daily task completion			
a. Has a plan for the day.			
b. Has a plan for the week.			
c. Initiates tasks on time.			
d. Avoids or overcomes distractions.			
e. Completes tasks on time.			
f. Stops (inhibits) tasks appropriately.			
6. Long-term projects			Identify project:
a. Plans appropriately for projects.			
At home			
At work			

(cont.)

Hierarchy of Skills	Yes	No	Comments
b. Completes projects.			
At home			
At work			
7. Is organized with respect to timely disposition and management of:			
a. Files and paperwork			
At home			
At work			
b. Clothes			
c. Mail			
d. Bill paying			
e. Laundry			
f. Meal preparation			
g. Dishwashing			
h. Other (specify) _____			
8. Emotional issues			
a. Denial of ADHD diagnosis			
b. Oppositionality/resistance to change			
c. Depression/demoralization			
d. Anxiety/fear of failure			
e. Perfectionism			

CHAPTER 6

Evidence Base
for Cognitive-Behavioral Therapy

DAVID J. MARKS

REVIEW OF COGNITIVE-BEHAVIORAL STUDIES

As noted in the preceding chapters, ADHD is a highly chronic psychiatric disorder that persists into adulthood in a substantial proportion of individuals and continues to exact a pernicious toll on multiple spheres of psychosocial functioning. As discussed in Chapter 1, even when effective, psychopharmacological interventions are often insufficient to address the deficits in time management, organization, and planning, as well as psychiatric comorbidities and dysfunctional automatic thoughts, and ingrained maladaptive behavior patterns that typically accompany ADHD in adults. The past decade has seen the emergence of CBT for adults with ADHD that are intended to address these important unmet clinical needs. In this chapter, I provide a review of the published literature in this area, as well as more detailed presentation of two studies from our research group that evaluated the outcomes of the treatment described in this book.

Relative to studies of psychosocial interventions in children, there is a dearth of investigations that have been undertaken to examine the effectiveness of psychosocial treatments for adults with ADHD. A search of the published literature yielded two individual case studies (Goodwin & Corgiat, 1992); five open-label, pre- and postevaluation studies of cognitive-behavioral interventions (Hesslinger et al., 2002; Solanto, Marks,

Mitchell, Wasserstein, & Kofman, 2008; Virta et al., 2008; Wiggins, Singh, Getz, & Hutchins, 1999; Wilens et al., 1999); three randomized controlled trials of CBT (Safren et al., 2005; Safren et al., 2010; Solanto et al., 2010; Stevenson, Whitmont, Bornholt, Livesey, & Stevenson, 2002); and a multimodal treatment program that included participation in individual CBT (Rostain & Ramsay, 2006).

McDermott and Wilens (2000) developed an individual CBT protocol that targeted dysfunctional cognitions believed to engender procrastination and avoidance. Therapeutic objectives included psychoeducation in cognitive distortions, monitoring and reevaluating of thought processes, and environmental restructuring (e.g., exposure to principles of scheduling and organization). According to a systematic chart review of 26 clients who participated in the program (mean number of sessions = 36), improvements were observed with respect to both ADHD symptoms as well as internalizing behaviors (Wilens et al., 1999). However, the fact that the vast majority of clients (85%) were receiving concomitant pharmacotherapy calls into question the extent to which treatment gains can be generalized to unmedicated adults.

Wiggins and colleagues (1999) compared a brief (four-session) group psychoeducational program, administered to nine participants, to a wait-list control sample of adults with ADHD ($n = 8$). Improvements were observed in the realms of organization (effect size of 1.7), attention (effect size of 1.9), and emotional stability (1.3). Some improvement was also observed in self-esteem, a finding that was attributable to heightened insight into the participants' perceived disability.

Using methods that draw conceptually on CBT fundamentals, Hesslinger and colleagues (2002) examined the efficacy of a 13-week group dialectical behavior therapy (DBT) program, which, in addition to psychoeducation (regarding both ADHD and depression), emphasized the following: mindfulness techniques, emotion regulation strategies (e.g., emotional record, diary cards), suppression of impulsivity (appreciating the consequences of dysregulation), stress management (problem solving and sequencing to alleviate anxiety), and the role of ADHD in relationships. Although treatment completers ($n = 8$) reported significantly greater reductions in depression, ADHD symptoms, and impairment relative to wait-list control participants ($n = 7$), small sample sizes in this study as well as the previous preclude definitive conclusions regarding efficacy and generalizability.

Stevenson and colleagues (2002) administered an eight-session cognitive remediation program to 22 adults with ADHD in weekly 2-hour sessions that focused on motivation, concentration, listening, impulsivity, organization, anger management, and self-esteem; the intervention incorporated both group treatment (to provide exposure to peer support) as well as individual coaching to ensure implementation, accountability, and individualization. Relative to those who participated in a wait-list control group ($n = 21$), participants assigned to cognitive remediation reported significant reductions in ADHD severity (effect size of 1.4) coupled with improvements in organization (effect size of 1.2). Based on their decrement in ADHD symptoms, 36% were considered responders immediately posttreatment; this increased to 55% two months after treatment discontinuation, however, initial improvements in self-esteem and anger management reportedly diminished. An examination of potential treatment moderators revealed that neither medication status nor internalizing disorders (anxiety or depression) impacted treatment outcomes.

Safren and colleagues (2005) conducted a clinical trial of a CBT program, administered in an individual modality, which comprised modules targeting organization and planning, distractibility, and cognitive restructuring; optional modules were also included that focused on procrastination, anger management, assertiveness training, and communication skills, for a maximum of 15 weekly sessions. Participants already receiving medication for ADHD were randomly assigned to receive either the addition of CBT ($n = 16$) or to continue on medication only ($n = 15$), and were evaluated at both baseline and posttreatment assessment points using independent evaluator and self-report measures of ADHD severity, anxiety, depression, and global functioning. Results indicated that those assigned to receive CBT experienced significantly greater reductions in independent-evaluator-reported and self-reported symptoms of ADHD and anxiety; also apparent was a significant diminution in independent-evaluator-rated depression along with a marginally significant decrease in self-reported depression. Using categorical estimates of treatment response, 56% of participants were classified as responders to the combined intervention compared with 13% for those assigned to continue on pharmacotherapy alone.

Using an exclusively multimodal design, Rostain and Ramsay (2006) examined the combined effectiveness of individual pharmacotherapy and cognitive-behavioral treatment in 43 adults with ADHD. Each participant received mixed amphetamine salts (Adderall) titrated up to 20 mg twice daily, with maintenance treatment provided for the best therapeutic dose; methylphenidate substitution was provided if deemed appropriate. The CBT program included sixteen 50-minute individual sessions that addressed psychoeducation, use of strength and support resources, instillation of more adaptive methods for coping with ADHD symptoms, and identification and modification of dysfunctional thoughts that underlie maladaptive coping and emotional disturbances (e.g., anxiety and depression). Significant reductions were observed in both self-reported and clinician-rated ADHD symptoms (Clinical Global Impression for ADHD [CGI-A]); 70% reported moderate to significant improvement in self-reported ratings, while 56% were found to be much or very much improved based on clinician ratings. In addition, significant improvements were demonstrated for self-reported and clinician-rated indices of depression and anxiety. Yet, despite the apparent benefits derived from treatment, the absence of a control group precluded efforts to differentiate the source of therapeutic gains (i.e., pharmacological vs. psychotherapeutic modalities).

More recently, Virta et al. (2008) evaluated the effectiveness of a 10- to 11-session group cognitive-behavioral rehabilitation program in 29 adults with ADHD (subtypes unspecified) using self-reported and collateral ratings (ADHD Checklist, BDI-II,

Symptom Checklist-90 [SCL-90], and the BADDS) obtained 3 months before treatment (T1), at the beginning of treatment (T2), and at the end of treatment (T3). Participants ranged in age between 18 and 45 years (median age = 31 years), and were evenly represented by men and women. Nineteen (66%) were taking stimulant medication for ADHD. Nine (31%) met diagnostic criteria for comorbid psychiatric disorder. Each 1½- to 2-hour session followed a structured sequence (i.e., review of the previous exercise, introduction of new thematic area, and introduction of the new exercise) and addressed themes considered by Brown (2008) to be central to ADHD (e.g., motivation and initiation of activities, organization, attention, emotional regulation, memory, impulsivity and psychiatric comorbidity, and self-esteem). Examination of self-report ratings indicated no significant differences between T1 and T2. In contrast, significant treatment effects (i.e., T2 vs. T3) were observed for self-reported activation, affect, and total subscales of the BADDS as well as items from the SCL-90 specifically relevant to ADHD symptoms. Using categorical estimates of response, more than 30% were reported to benefit from the treatment (> 20% decrease in symptoms) based on self-reported measures. However, the absence of a control or comparison group constrained efforts to gauge the effectiveness of this program.

Finally, Safren and colleagues (Safren et al., 2010) recently completed a randomized controlled trial examining the effectiveness of individual CBT for medicated adults with ADHD who continued to display clinically significant symptoms. CBT comprised the same core modules administered in their previous study (Safren et al., 2005). Eighty-seven adults were randomized to receive either CBT or a comparison treatment consisting of relaxation training with psychoeducation. Results indicated that a significantly greater proportion of individuals assigned to CBT (vs. comparison) were classified as treatment responders on the basis of blind clinician ratings on the Clinical Global Index (CGI) and the ADHD Rating Scale (ADHD-RS) (CGI: 53% vs. 23%; ADHD-RS: 67% vs. 33%). Analogous findings were observed using self-reported ratings.

STUDIES OF THE MOUNT SINAI CBT PROGRAM FOR ADHD*

Based upon the seemingly ubiquitous deficiencies in time-management, organization, and planning skills among adults with ADHD, our group developed the CBT program, described in the Treatment Manual, that draws heavily from behavioral and cognitive-

---

*We had originally titled our treatment "metacognitive therapy," and this term was used in our first two papers (Solanto et al., 2008, 2010). However, it was noted that this term conflicts with the use of the term as originated by Adrian Wells (2005) to describe a quite different type of therapy. While we use the term metacognitive therapy (MCT) in this section where we describe the results of our two studies, we otherwise refer, as we have previously and will henceforth refer, to our treatment simply as cognitive-behavioral therapy for adult ADHD.

behavioral principles and is designed to provide training in specific skills, reinforce and shape positive behavior, substitute more adaptive cognitions, and challenge maladaptive self-statements. As noted previously, sessions are typically implemented in groups of six to eight persons and incorporate exposure to didactic techniques, in-session modeling and rehearsal of metacognitive strategies, identification and reconciliation of obstacles to progress (e.g., cognitive distortions), and dissemination of Take-Home Exercises to reinforce key concepts.

Open Trial

As part of a preliminary investigation, 38 adults (16 men, 22 women) with ADHD participated in either 8- or 12-week iterations of the manualized group program (Solanto et al., 2008). Participants ranged in age from 23 to 65 years (M [SD]) age = 41.82 [9.98] years) and met criteria for either ADHD, combined type (n = 14; 36.8%), or ADHD, predominantly inattentive type (n = 24; 63.2%). The diagnosis of ADHD was confirmed for all individuals on the basis of a comprehensive clinical interview along with the Conners' Adult ADHD Rating Scales—Self-Report: Long Form (CAARS-S:L; Conners et al., 1999). Individuals with a T-score ≥ 65 (clinical range) on the DSM-IV inattentive symptoms scale and < 65 on the DSM-IV hyperactive–impulsive symptoms scale were classified as having ADHD, predominantly inattentive type; those with T-scores ≥ 65 on both subscales were categorized as ADHD, combined type. Participants were well educated and of middle- to upper-middle socioeconomic status. Twenty-six (68.4%) were concomitantly receiving psychotropic medication for ADHD. Approximately 58% of participants were noted to meet criteria for a comorbid mood disorder, while 39.5% met criteria for a coexisting anxiety disorder. Individuals with significant anger-management disturbances, current psychoactive substance abuse or dependence, or serious mental health problems (e.g., suicidality) were excluded from participation.

Thirty adults (79%) completed the program, 21 (70%) of whom were concurrently receiving psychostimulant medication for ADHD. Individuals who did and did not complete the program did not differ with regard to demographic variables (e.g., age, socioeconomic status, ethnicity, education level), baseline severity of ADHD, medication status, or rates of internalizing disorder comorbidity. In addition, those who were and were not taking medication for ADHD did not differ with respect to baseline severity of ADHD, presence or absence of an internalizing disorder, or ADHD subtype.

Both abbreviated (8-session) and expanded (12-session) group programs were co-led by two psychologists and incorporated identical treatment principles (with the latter allowing for more graduated exposure to therapeutic techniques). All participants completed the following self-report behavioral rating scales immediately prior to and following the completion of the program to gauge their response to the MCT intervention:

1. CAARS-S:L, a psychometrically sound, 66-item self-report inventory that assesses core features of ADHD (i.e., DSM-IV inattentive, hyperactive–impulsive, and total symptoms) as well as associated behavioral features (Conners et al., 1999).
2. BAADS (Brown, 1996), a 40-item self-report questionnaire designed to gauge proficiency in six domains of executive functioning (i.e., organization and prioritization, focused and sustained attention, regulation of alertness and sustained effort, affect modulation, working memory, and self-regulation) as well as overall executive function abilities.
3. ON-TOP, a 24-item self-report inventory developed within our program to assess perceived competencies in the realms of time-management, organization, and planning skills (possible score range: –102 to +102).

As shown in Table 6.1, MCT yielded significant posttreatment decreases in DSM-IV-TR inattention symptoms and composite and individual domain scores from the BAADS, as well as the total score from the ON-TOP. Although no significant decrease was observed in self-reported DSM-IV hyperactive–impulsive symptoms, it should be emphasized that such behaviors were not in the clinical range prior to treatment and were not formally targeted by the intervention. Further examination of pre–post group CAARS-S:L DSM-IV inattentive symptom ratings revealed that 46.7% of participants decreased from the clinical range (T-score ≥ 65) to below the clinical threshold (T-score

TABLE 6.1. Pre- and Posttreatment Scores on ADHD Scales in Open Trial

	Mean (SD)			
	Pretreatment	Posttreatment	p	Effect size[a]
CAARS-S:L DSM-IV subscales				
Inattentive Symptoms	83.26 (8.37)	68.52 (14.86)	.000	0.588
Hyperactive–Impulsive Symptoms	59.00 (14.12)	54.67 (13.57)	NS	
BADDS subscales				
Total Score	82.74 (7.98)	67.44 (11.26)	.000	0.669
Activation	83.83 (7.24)	70.45 (11.54)	.000	0.595
Attention	74.62 (9.85)	63.59 (10.32)	.000	0.558
Effort	84.76 (10.53)	66.24 (15.59)	.000	0.591
Affect	68.90 (10.31)	59.62 (9.75)	.000	0.449
Memory	75.24 (11.21)	64.86 (8.54)	.000	0.527
ON-TOP	–43.70 (24.73)	–16.48 (24.12)	.000	0.615

Note. From Solanto, Marks, Mitchell, Wasserstein, and Kofman (2008). Copyright 2008 by Sage Publications, Inc. Reprinted by permission.
[a]Partial eta-squared.

< 65), a pattern that was not impacted by medication status. Finally, pre–post scores did not appear to be appreciably impacted by initial depression severity.

It was therefore inferred that the MCT treatment program yields acute reductions in self-reported ADHD severity and executive dysfunction, and holds promise as an effective treatment modality for adults with ADHD. It was particularly noteworthy that incremental benefits occurred despite that more than half of those who completed the program were receiving pharmacotherapy. When juxtaposed with the fact that medicated and unmedicated participants did not differ with respect to initial ADHD severity, this finding suggests that there is room for improvement even among adults medicated for ADHD.

Randomized Controlled Trial

Despite the apparent short-term benefits of MCT, the preliminary investigation did not control for expectancy of change and spontaneous diminution of symptoms over time, nor did it take into account the nonspecific effects of therapy (e.g., mutual support and information sharing). In addition, the imposition of a fee for treatment may have resulted in a less representative (e.g., better educated and more functional) client base that may have been better able to assimilate and/or implement treatment principles.

On the basis of the above findings and methodological constraints, it was hypothesized that more robust therapeutic change would occur to individuals receiving MCT versus a supportive psychotherapy group that controlled for nonspecific therapeutic elements. In addition, it was hypothesized that, by improving daily functioning, MCT (vs. supportive psychotherapy) would reduce comorbid symptoms of anxiety and depression. Finally, despite the absence of effects of medication in the small open trial, it was hypothesized that medication would interact with the treatment group, such that MCT participants taking medication would better assimilate the treatment techniques and more successfully apply the interventions between sessions and thereby achieve better outcomes.

To test the above predictions, we pursued and acquired National Institute of Mental Health (NIMH) funding to undertake a randomized clinical trial of group MCT (Solanto et al., 2010). For this study, 88 adults rigorously diagnosed with ADHD (see diagnostic procedures below) were stratified with respect to use or non-use of ADHD medications (psychostimulants or atomoxetine) and randomly assigned to either a 12-week group MCT program (n = 45) or a 12-week supportive psychotherapy group (n = 43); the latter was comparable to the MCT program with regard to session length and number of participants (approximately six to eight per group) and was designed to control for nonspecific aspects of treatment (e.g., therapist psychoeducation and group support). Response was assessed via a structured interview completed by an independent (blind) evaluator and by questionnaires completed by the participant and a collateral informant immediately pre- and posttreatment. MCT and supportive psychotherapy groups were run in yoked cohorts to ensure that the conditions were equivalent with regard to environmental changes (e.g., seasonal and holiday periods). A total of six cohort waves were conducted, with each therapist (D.J.M. and J.W.) leading an equal number of MCT and supportive psycho-therapy groups.

As with the earlier pilot investigation, participants were required to be between the ages of 18 and 65 with a diagnosis of ADHD (predominantly inattentive or combined type) and were excluded on the basis of the following criteria: active substance abuse or dependence, suicidality, asocial characteristics (e.g., pervasive developmental disor-der), cognitive disability (estimated Full Scale IQ < 80), borderline personality disorder, Alzheimer's disease or suspected dementia, childhood history of trauma or other severe psychiatric disorder that confounded the determination of childhood ADHD symptoms, and/or the presence of acute psychiatric disturbance(s) considered to represent the essen-tial focus of clinical attention. Clients were admonished to defer modifications to their medication and/or psychosocial treatment regimens until the end of treatment.

The diagnosis of ADHD was determined using the CAADID for DSM-IV (Epstein et al., 2001) along with a T-score ≥ 65 (93rd percentile) on the CAARS-S:L DSM-IV inattentive subscale and a). In addition, potential candidates were required to show impairment (T-score ≥ 63, equal to the 90th percentile on the CAARS-S:L inattention/ memory subscale [CAARS-IN], which contains a predominance of items relevant to time management, organization, and planning). The presence of childhood ADHD symptoms was validated by at least one of the following: self-report of four or more childhood symp-toms in one domain on the CAADID, collateral report using the Childhood Symptom Scale—Other Report (Barkley & Murphy, 1998), or reports of symptoms on a school report or a childhood psychological evaluation. Concurrent psychiatric comorbidity was assessed using the Structured Clinical Interview for DSM-IV Axis I Disorders (SCID-I; First, Spitzer, Gibbon, & Williams, 2002) and the SCID-II module for borderline person-ality disorder (First, Gibbon, Spitzer, Williams, & Benjamin, 1997). IQ was estimated using four subtests from the WAIS-III, using a procedure outlined by Tellegen and Briggs (1967).

Participants were assessed by the independent evaluator pre- and posttreatment using the Adult ADHD Investigator Symptom Rating Scale (AISRS; Adler, Spencer, & Bieder-man, 2003), which is a structured clinical interview designed to gauge the presence and severity of the 18 DSM-IV symptoms of ADHD. The independent evaluator also admin-istered the Structured Interview Guide for the Hamilton Anxiety Rating Scale (SIGH-A; Shear et al., 2001). The total symptom score, summed across the nine AISRS inattention items (AISRS-IN) and the CAARS-IN subscale served as the primary outcome mea-sures. In addition, the following questionnaires were completed pre- and posttreatment: CAARS—Observer Report; BAADS; BRIEF-A (Roth et al., 2005); BDI-II (Beck, Steer, & Brown, 1996); Rosenberg Self-Esteem Inventory (Rosenberg, 1965); and the ON-TOP.

Similarly to the initial study, the MCT group employed behavioral and cognitive-behavioral principles to provide contingent self-reward, dismantle complex tasks into manageable elements, sustain motivation, and challenge anxiogenic and depressogenic cognitions. As discussed in earlier chapters, the program was hierarchical in design such that exposure to basic principles (e.g., mechanics of planner use) preceded exposure to higher-order skills (e.g., organization and planning). Concerted efforts were made to link problematic situations (cues) to explicit solutions and to identify obstacles to successful implementation.

The supportive psychotherapy group was developed to control for nonspecific components of the MCT program, including session and treatment duration, group support/validation, therapist attention, and psychoeducation, yet precluded the discussion or endorsement of cognitive-behavioral principles. Across all iterations of the program, the support group was characterized as a mechanism for providing information (e.g., addressing and dispelling myths), uniting around common experiences, and engendering collaborative support. Each session was divided into two distinct segments, with the initial half devoted to a review of events that transpired during the previous week, and the second to a therapist-led discussion of a specific psychoeducational theme. Throughout the various sessions, the therapist responded by offering support and encouragement and/or by referring the concern to the group for alternative solutions.

With the exception of marital status (i.e., greater proportion of currently married participants in MCT vs. supportive psychotherapy), MCT and supportive psychotherapy participants did not differ with regard to sociodemographic or clinical variables. As shown in Table 6.2, general linear modeling (GLM) analyses, comparing change from baseline between treatment groups, revealed significant effects for independent-evaluator measures of inattention (AISRS-IN) and time-management, organizational and planning skills (AISRS-TMOP) as well as collateral ratings on the inattention/memory subscale (CAARS-IN-Observer). Stated differently, the decrement in severity from pre- to posttest periods, controlling for initial ratings, was more robust for individuals assigned to MCT. For other measures of executive function, an examination of confidence intervals revealed significant change from pre- to posttreatment for supportive psychotherapy as well as MCT; however, the change score difference *between groups* was not significant (BADDS) or only marginally significant (BRIEF Metacognitive Index, ON-TOP). Measures of comorbidity (depression, anxiety, self-esteem) revealed no significant change in either treatment. Only one statistically significant interaction was observed between baseline score and response to treatment: the larger (more severe) the CAARS-IN score at baseline, the greater the differential improvement with MCT; change in the supportive psychotherapy group, by contrast, was stable across the entire range of initial CAARS-IN scores.

Dichotomous indices of therapeutic response were also examined to determine whether participants exhibited a clinically meaningful response to treatment. On the AISRS, a positive response was operationalized as a decrease of 30%; positive response on the CAARS-IN was defined as a decrease of ≥ 10 T-score points (1 *SD*). Using the aforementioned criteria, a significantly greater proportion of MCT participants were classified as responders versus supportive psychotherapy participants (42% and 12%, respectively).

TABLE 6.2. Response to MCT and Support Group Treatments on Dimensional Measures

Measure	MCT group (n = 41)								Support group (n = 40)								Difference between least squares mean change scores (95% CI)
	Pre		Post		Least squares mean change[a]	(95% CI)			Pre		Post		Least squares mean change	(95% CI)			
	Mean	(SD)	Mean	(SD)					Mean	(SD)	Mean	(SD)					
AISRS-IN	18.88	(3.75)	13.71	(4.27)	5.0	(3.7, 6.3)*			18.33	(3.55)	16.18	(4.71)	2.3	(1.0, 3.6)*			2.7 (0.9, 4.6)***
AISRS-TMOP	10.98	(2.30)	7.66	(2.83)	3.2	(2.3, 4.1)*			10.58	(2.59)	9.70	(3.16)	1.0	(0.1, 1.9)*			2.2 (0.9, 3.5)****
Conners-Observer-IN[b,c]	72.47	(10.56)	66.94	(11.64)	5.7	(3.1, 8.3)*			74.33	(9.67)	73.19	(10.33)	0.9	(-2.0, 3.9)			4.8 (0.8, 8.7)*
BADDS total T-score	84.73	(8.82)	75.80	(12.63)	9.1	(6.0, 12.2)*			85.72	(9.53)	76.80	(11.00)	8.8	(5.6, 12.0)*			0.3 (-4.2, 4.7)
BRIEF-A Metacognitive Index[c]	78.37	(8.69)	73.83	(9.01)	5.39	(2.2, 8.6)*			80.71	(9.24)	78.64	(11.52)	1.26	(-2.0, 4.6)			4.13 (-0.5, 8.7)+
ON-TOP	-40.56	(23.87)	-22.10	(20.64)	-17.9	(-23.7, -2.1)*			-37.87	(22.57)	-28.98	(24.67)	-9.5	(-15.5, -3.4)*			-8.4 (-16.8, 0.0)+
BDI-II	11.48	(9.59)	9.66	(8.31)	1.8	(-0.1, 3.7)			11.34	(8.12)	9.08	(7.16)	2.3	(0.3, 4.3)*			-0.5 (-3.2, 2.2)
Hamilton—total anxiety	9.56	(5.37)	8.07	(5.38)	1.2	(-0.2, 2.7)			8.45	(5.20)	8.88	(5.63)	-0.2	(-1.7, 1.3)			1.4 (-0.7, 3.5)
Hamilton—observed anxiety[d]	0.65	(0.74)	0.50	(0.64)	0.2	(-0.0, 0.3)			0.50	(0.64)	0.65	(0.70)	-0.1	(-0.3, 0.1)			0.3 (-0.0, 0.5)
Rosenberg Self-Esteem Inventory	16.93	(5.14)	18.39	(6.02)	-1.3	(-2.6, 0.0)			18.37	(5.62)	19.50	(5.86)	-1.3	(-2.7, 0.1)			-0.0 (-1.9, 1.9)

Note. AISRS, Adult ADHD Investigator Symptom Rating Scale (blind structured interview; IN, inattentive symptoms; TMOP, symptoms relating to time management, organization, and planning); Conners-Observer-IN, Conners Adult ADHD Rating Scales—Observer: Long Form, Inattention/Memory subscale; BADDS, Brown ADD Scales; BRIEF-A, Behavior Rating Inventory of Executive Function—Adult Version; ON-TOP, On Time Management, Organization, and Planning Scale (range of scores for ON-TOP is -102 to +102); BDI-II, Beck Depression Inventory—Second Edition; Hamilton, Hamilton Anxiety Rating Scale. Scores for CAARS, BADDS, and BRIEF are T-scores. From Solanto et al. (2010). Copyright by the American Psychiatric Association. Reprinted by permission.

[a]Least squares mean change is change from baseline (pre minus post) adjusted for baseline value.

[b]MCT n = 34; support n = 27.

[c]The difference between groups was no longer significant (Conners-Observer-IN) or no longer approached significance (BRIEF-A) after excluding noncompleters and medication changers.

[d]This refers to anxiety observed and rated by the interviewer during the structured interview.

+*p* < .10; *p* < .05; **p* < .01; ***p* < .005; ****p* < .001.

A statistically significant difference in response rate was also observed using self-report (CAARS-IN) ratings (53% and 28%, respectively). Thus, while indicators of change for the primary outcome measures clearly favored the MCT group, it is important to emphasize that individuals assigned to the supportive psychotherapy group also derived appreciable benefit.

Contrary to expectations, minimal differences were observed between treatment groups with regard to changes in scores for depression (BDI-II), self-esteem (Rosenberg), or anxiety (SIGH-A). Apart from a small but statistically significant reduction in depression (BDI-II) scores for supportive psychotherapy, no significant group effects were observed for any comorbidity outcome measure. Although the specific reason(s) why MCT did not more appreciably impact measures of comorbidity is unclear, the fact that baseline scores on these measures did not fall within the clinical range points to the possibility of floor effects.

Additional analyses indicated no significant difference between groups vis-à-vis expectancy ratings obtained pretreatment or after the first two treatment sessions. Moreover, age, gender, ethnicity, education, household income, marital status, employment status, IQ, ADHD subtype, concurrent medication for ADHD, and presence of a comorbid mood and/or anxiety disorder did not interact with the effects of treatment; in each analysis, the effect of MCT versus supportive psychotherapy remained significant while controlling for each of the above variables, and in no case did they interact with the effect of treatment. However, within the MCT group, completion of the Take-Home Exercise was significantly related to change in AISRS-IN score, highlighting the importance of this treatment component.

Several factors may have accounted for why medication did not interact with the treatment group to moderate treatment response. First, the fact that participants were required to meet entry criteria for minimum levels of symptom severity may have oversampled for nonresponders or suboptimal responders to medication. This may be especially likely given that medicated and nonmedicated participants did not differ with respect to baseline levels of ADHD severity. Although analyses were conducted using a subset of participants considered to be adequately medicated, it is conceivable that specific medication(s) and dosage(s) may not have been optimally titrated by individual practitioners. A final possibility, and one that is consistent with findings from our initial investigation of primarily medicated participants (Solanto et al., 2008), is that the MCT intervention is sufficiently structured for participants to benefit irrespective of medication status.

SUMMARY AND CONCLUSIONS

To date, five uncontrolled, four randomized controlled trials, and a multimodal treatment program have been undertaken to examine the efficacy of cognitive-behavioral interventions for the treatment of adult ADHD; however, only the study described immediately above (Solanto et al., 2010), and the recently completed study by Safren (Safren et al., 2010) controlled for nonspecific treatment elements. As demonstrated by the above studies, cognitive-behavioral treatment, delivered in individual or group modalities, in the presence or absence of psychopharmacological intervention, can help to mitigate the core features of ADHD (i.e., inattention), associated impairments in executive skills (e.g., time-management, organization, and planning skills), and for some, the severity of comorbid anxiety and depression symptoms. It therefore appears that many adults with ADHD can benefit from explicit training in self-management techniques, either to compensate for their absence/immaturity, or to provide heightened levels of accountability and motivation.

Despite the acute benefits conferred by such interventions, it remains as yet unresolved the extent to which treatment-related benefits are maintained beyond the point of treatment termination. In addition, future studies would be well served to consider the use of a multifactorial (e.g., 2×2) design to rigorously gauge the independent and combined effects of optimally titrated pharmacotherapy and psychosocial treatments for the management of ADHD in adults. Such a design may also enable investigators to determine the moderator variables (e.g., initial ADHD severity, comorbidity) associated with preferential response to individual or combined treatment modalities.

In conclusion, given the active interest on the part of clinicians, researchers, and those directly affected by ADHD, and given as well recent innovations in intervention, the future looks promising for the continued development of psychosocial treatments to treat the deficits associated with adult ADHD.

TREATMENT MANUAL

Introduction for Therapists

This Treatment Manual is a session-by-session guide to a 12-session treatment program designed to foster the development of time-management, organizational, and planning skills in adults with ADHD. Each session has Leader Notes, as well as Take-Home Notes and a Take-Home Exercise to be distributed to the participants.

STRUCTURE AND FORMAT OF THE MANUAL

The Leader Notes are intended to highlight the principles and strategies to be presented and discussed at each meeting. They are not intended to be delivered strictly as a script but rather to provide an outline of the material to be covered, along with suggested phrasing of material for greatest clarity and maximum impact upon group participants. Material that is important for the therapist to specifically articulate is presented in **bold and italics** and may be given verbatim. In general, however, the style of the group should remain interactive rather than expository during the presentation portion, as well as during the review of the Take-Home Exercise. Thus, group participants may pose questions or raise issues during the presentation to which the therapist may respond by using them as opportunities to explain the concepts and strategies planned for the session.

The Take-Home Notes are intended to provide a pithy review, recapitulation, and reemphasis of the material covered in the session. In some cases, additional suggestions are provided that may not have been covered in the sessions. The Take-Home Notes are intended to compensate for possible lapses of attention in the session and also to set the stage for the Take-Home Exercise. They provide a valuable tool for future reference and review and should be sent out to individuals who miss the session. An optional, but helpful, tactic is to send out an e-mail to all members midway between sessions to bolster motivation and encourage completion of the Take-Home Exercises.

Scattered through the Leader Notes are a few "Notes to Therapists" in which we highlight an issue or concern that is typically voiced by participants in response to the material presented in that session, and suggest how the therapist may address that concern.

Material concerning selection of patients for group treatment and a discussion of style of delivery of treatment may be found in Chapter 3 of the Therapist Guide.

FORMAT OF GROUP SESSIONS

The program is designed for a group of six to eight adults meeting weekly for 2 hours over 12 weeks. Our groups are scheduled in the evening, 6:30 to 8:30, so as to allow working adults to complete the workday, have dinner, and travel to the session. The format of each group session is as follows:

1. Review of Take-Home Exercise (up to 1 hour).
2. Presentation and discussion of new material (45 minutes, including In-Session Exercise).
3. In-Session Exercise.
4. Presentation and discussion of next Take-Home Exercise (15 minutes).

OPTIONAL SESSIONS

The following sessions were not included in our formal efficacy study published in 2010, but we have since found it helpful to schedule one or both of the following, thereby expanding the Group program to 13 or 14 sessions: an additional session for the material on automatic thoughts and cognitive distortions, and a session concerning "Getting to Bed, Getting Up, and Getting to Work on Time." The additional session on automatic thoughts divides the material in the current Session 5 into two sessions—one on identifying cognitive distortions, and one on challenging them. This arrangement allows participants more time to assimilate this material. The break points to be used for the presentation and Take-Home Exercise are indicated in Session 5. The additional material on "Getting to Bed, Getting Up, and Getting to Work on Time" is relevant for some, but not all persons with ADHD and is included at the end of the manual. Querying about this during the screening visit for the group will reveal how many potential group participants have difficulty in this area.

LEADER NOTES

Making Peace with the Diagnosis and Committing to Growth

Introduction to Goals and Methods of the Group

Goals:
- Orient participants to the methods and expectations of the group.
- Help participants identify their:
  - Personal goals for the group.
  - Emotions that may produce resistance to change.
  - Inner resources that they may draw upon to facilitate change.

New Target Skills:

Regular and prompt **attendance** and **completion and storage of Take Home Exercise**.

Take-Home Exercise:

Written reflection on making peace with the diagnosis and committing to growth.

NOTE TO THERAPIST: Before the start of the session proper, be sure the participants have completed any questionnaires (e.g., CAARS, BRIEF, ON-TOP, Beck) that may be desirable to use to assess improvement as a result of group treatment. Then begin the session by introducing yourself and going around the room, asking each group member to introduce him- or herself and share a bit about what he or she does, his or her diagnosis of ADHD, and what he or she is hoping to achieve in the group. Then present the following:

I. METHODS OF THE GROUP THERAPY PROGRAM

The program is described as "cognitive-behavioral" in nature, because some components aim to change behavior while others aim to change cognitions.

Behavioral

An example of a behavioral strategy taught in the program is to use a planner to enter all appointments and tasks, and to check the planner at regular intervals. Another example is to reward oneself after completing a particularly difficult or tedious task or project.

Cognitive

Cognitions are thoughts in the form of self-instructions that we use to guide ourselves through the day. Cognitions can also be the thoughts—or "self-talk"—we have about ourselves and our abilities. The program aims to:

1. **Instill more adaptive self-instructions,** such as:
   "I will plan to complete this large project by dividing it into smaller, more manageable parts."
2. **Challenge negative self-talk,** such as:
   "I never do anything right."
   "I *should* be able to work at top efficiency for the entire day."
   "Everything in my life is a mess and will never get better."
   and substitute more positive cognitions, such as:
   "It doesn't have to be perfect—just good enough."
   "I usually do better than I fear."
   "There are many things I can do well."

The goal here is to address the **emotional** obstacles to success and satisfaction.

Cognitive-Behavioral Synergy

The cognitive and behavioral components of the program work to enhance each other: More efficient and organized behavior helps to establish more positive cognitions about ourselves. More adaptive cognitions generate more positive behavior, which in turn creates and sustains more positive cognitions about ourselves and about future possibilities.

II. FORMAT OF EACH SESSION

Each session consists of the following:

1. **Review of previous week's progress and Take-Home Exercise.** Clarify that Take-Home Exercises will be handed out weekly and they will not be handed in. They are for the participant to keep and to discuss with the

group as desired. Also recommend that participants keep their homework/ binder in a private place to ensure the information cannot be read by others.

2. **Presentation of new material, with discussion and in-session exercise.**
3. **Presentation of next Take-Home Exercise, with anticipatory troubleshooting.**

Working through the Take-Home Exercise will have more impact than anything else on how much you benefit from the group program. Note that the strategies introduced one by one in the Take-Home Exercises are intended to be cumulative; that is, once you have completed the exercise—say, prioritizing the tasks for a week—it is hoped that you will continue to practice and utilize that strategy in your daily life.

If you have difficulty completing the Take-Home Exercise, or even if you do not complete it at all, don't let that keep you from coming to the session (out of guilt/shame, etc.). It's expected that you will have some difficulty—and those are the very problems we will want to discuss at the next session.

III. GROUND RULES

1. **Regular and on-time attendance.** Stress the importance of *commitment* to self and to the group. ***Others are depending on your support and input. The group will be less successful without you. Call if you won't be able to come.*** Take time here to address any obvious or potential problems with on-time attendance of any group member(s).
2. **Confidentiality.** *What is said here stays here.*
3. **Treatment changes.** *If you make any changes to your treatment regimen—for example, starting, stopping, or changing dose or type of medication, or starting/stopping psychotherapy, please let us know so we can better assess your progress in the group.*

IV. COMMITMENT

Highlight the need for commitment to the program and importance of completing the Take-Home Exercises. ***People with ADHD can become experts at time management—perhaps even more so than the average person—because they will have made it a special focus/challenge and worked at it.***

Making changes—doing things differently—may seem strange at first. It may seem as though you are having to "force yourself," which may feel "unnatural." Or you may feel anxious about not "doing it right." These are NOT indi-

cations that you should stop. Rather, it means you should keep pushing through until the new habits seem more easy and natural—and over time they will!

Questions and Answers about ADHD

Open the floor to any questions participants may have about ADHD, its diagnosis, or its treatment.

V. Pass Out Copies of the Session-by-Session Plan for the Group Program

VI. Compile a List of E-Mail Addresses

The therapist needs to communicate with group participants easily should there be a change in the schedule (e.g., due to weather), and in order to send materials to any member who has missed a session. Obtain the permission of each group member to have his or her e-mail address shared with the others to facilitate communication among participants outside the session.

VII. Take-Home Exercise: Making Peace with the Diagnosis and Committing to Growth

Pass out and discuss the Take-Home Exercise.

1. Introduce the group to the purpose and content of the exercise.
   - To gain insights into where group participants might now "be" in terms of accepting/working through the diagnosis and preparing to make changes.
2. Work through with the group *when* each member will complete the Take-Home Exercise.
   - When/how they would usually complete such a task (e.g., at the last minute? on the subway en route to the session?).
   - Discuss the pros and cons of different approaches to completion. Do anticipatory troubleshooting regarding procrastination, forgetting, and so on.
   - Insofar as possible, have each group member commit to a day, time, and place to complete the exercise.
3. Instruct group members to get a three-ring binder (½" thick) in which to store Take-Home Notes and Take-Home Exercises and bring to each session. Work through *where* each member will store the binder with homework and program information.
4. Ask each member of the group to bring to the next meeting the planners, address book, and to-do lists that he or she currently uses.

TAKE-HOME EXERCISE

Making Peace with the Diagnosis and Committing to Growth

I. INTRODUCTION

You've been diagnosed with ADHD. You may have suspected it or it may come as somewhat of a surprise to you. Your feelings may be very mixed at this point.

- There may be *relief* at finally having a problem recognized and labeled for what it is—a valid medical condition, *which is not now, and never was, your "fault."*
- There may be renewed *hope* that help may be available to you.
- You may still have many *questions* about ADHD—many of which I hope we will be able to answer here.
- You may still be in *doubt* about the diagnosis.
- You may *dislike* the idea that you have a condition that affects the way you think and act.
- You may be *angry* that this condition wasn't recognized and treated a long time ago, and that you suffered because of it.

What feeling or combination of feelings are you experiencing about this now?

_____

_____

II. MOVING ON

The fact that you're here says that you want to move on and grow; that you want to learn how to cope with the effects of this disorder and make some positive changes in your life. So let's begin there.

(cont.)

What are the reasons you decided to come for treatment now?

_____

_____

_____

III. COMMITTING TO CHANGE

However motivated we may be, contemplating making changes in our lives can feel risky, with both pros and cons. Check those that apply.

Possible Pros:

___ Less depression, increased optimism

___ Feelings of being "in charge"

___ Positive feedback from others

___ Enhanced self-esteem and self-efficacy

Possible Cons:

___ Risky/unknown

___ Not comfortable

___ Fears of failing yet again

___ Uncertainty about how others will react

IV. DEALING WITH OLD HURTS/ANGERS/ADDRESSING THE PAST

What was the hardest thing for you about having ADHD as a child?

_____

_____

_____

(cont.)

What would you say now to help a child with ADHD?

_____

_____

_____

What would you say to your best friend if he or she had ADHD (now as an adult)?

_____

_____

_____

V. IDENTIFYING STRENGTHS/INTERNAL RESOURCES

We all have untapped resources that can help in overcoming obstacles. Having had ADHD may have had *positive* effects for you in this regard. Having had to cope with adversities often causes individuals to develop inner *strengths* of resourcefulness, perseverance, and determination. Other characteristics you may have developed to help you cope may include a sense of humor, friendliness, compassion, and so on.

What positive qualities do you feel you have developed as a result of having to struggle with ADHD?

_____

_____

_____

LEADER NOTES

Time Management

Time Awareness and Scheduling

New Target Skills:
- Constant access to timepieces (watches, clocks).
- Time estimation.
- Selection/purchase of planner.
- Use of planner for to-do lists and scheduling.

In-Session Exercise:
- Discuss pros and cons of various types of planners.

Take-Home Exercise:
- Evaluate personal planner.
- Time estimation.
- Time log.

I. REVIEW OF TAKE-HOME EXERCISE

Here the emphasis is less on the content of the task but **primarily on how the participants actually planned for and completed the home exercise**. Inquire about **whether** individuals scheduled the task, **when** they actually completed it, and **how** optimal the process was. Be alert for such problems as failing to allocate time, underestimating the time required, or failing to follow through on allocated time, as well as avoidance of, or anxiety concerning, the task itself (e.g., fears of failure). Consider the possible reasons for each of these, including oppositionality, defeatism, performance anxiety, and so on.

Allow participants to share as much as they want concerning the actual content of the exercise, particularly any insights they may have gained as a result of doing it.

Issues/problems discussed above can easily be used to segue into the following presentation/discussion.

II. TIME AWARENESS

Research indicates that people with ADHD have more difficulty in tracking the passage of time and adjusting their activities accordingly. They tend to make more errors in estimating how long things take and therefore may not allow sufficient time to complete chores, homework, office work, projects, and so on. Some of these errors may reflect "wishful thinking"—that is, the belief that a tedious or boring task (such as paying bills) can be completed in a shorter period of time than is realistic.

This indicates the need for people with ADHD to develop better awareness of time through the following:

1. Need to wear a watch, and have clocks clearly visible at all times in the home and in the office.
2. Need to estimate and then actually time **how long everyday tasks** require.

NOTE TO THERAPIST: **Ask how many in the group are actually wearing watches at the moment. You're likely to find that many are not.** Inquire of those not wearing a watch why they are not. One reason typically given is "I don't need it—I can use my cell phone." **(Response: One can't easily and quickly check the time on a cell phone, and one needs to be able to do so in order to become more "time aware.")** It is often the case that adults with ADHD have had a "love–hate" relationship with time and do not *want* to know how much time is passing. However, they cannot learn to master time without a watch.

III. SELECTION AND USE OF PLANNER

Ask participants to show the type of planner, to-do lists, and address book they currently use.

Planner Selection

Present alternative types of paper and digital planners and the pros and cons of each. Paper planners, such as Filofax, may be better for those who are not computer savvy and visual. Digital planners allow easy scheduling of repeating events, changes in appointments or tasks, and transfer of items on to-do lists. Digital planners may be more compact and neater. It is essential that the planner be easily portable, and that it have ample space for daily to-do lists.

"Commandments" of Planner Use

1. ***Thou may have one planner and one planner only.*** You must choose one planner; commit to it and stick with it.

2. ***Thou must carry thy planner with thee at all times.*** The planner must be portable and you must have it with you at all times to check appointment times, enter items to do, and so on. If you run into someone on the street and the opportunity arises to schedule an appointment you want to have your planner available.

3. ***Thou shalt enter every appointment and task into thy planner!*** This is when one makes the commitment to completing the appointment or the task. Unless and until it is entered into the planner, it docs not exist and therefore surely will not get done!

4. ***Thou shalt consult thy planner every morning, every midday, and every evening! (In other words, you may not start your day without a plan!)*** What's in the planner will have no impact on your life unless you consult it regularly—as regularly as you brush your teeth. It must become a thrice-daily habit. You consult it at night to make plans for the morning for travel, wardrobe, office materials, and so on that you need to bring the next day. You consult it in the morning to remind yourself of what is scheduled for the day so as to "hit the ground running" as the day begins and to ensure that nothing is forgotten. You need to consult it at midday to revise and reprioritize the activities for the afternoon, given the events of the morning. ***At least once a day, you must update the planner and reschedule the uncompleted items. Set a "cue" for yourself to remember to check your planner—for example, when you're making your coffee in the morning, during your lunch break, and when you're setting your alarm clock at night.***

REMEMBER: *If it's not in the planner, it doesn't exist!*

IV. USING TO-DO LISTS

1. Set up regular weekly time slots for recurring "functions" in your work week—for example, report/memo writing, calling clients, meetings, work in the field, and so on. The total amount of time per week that you need to allocate to each of these functions will become clearer after you complete the time log (Take-Home Exercise).

2. Set up to-do lists corresponding to each of your main projects, clients, accounts, and so on. For example, if you work on Projects A, B, and C, you would have separate lists of items that need to be done for each of these projects. When the time allocated in your planner arrives to work for that client or project, consult the appropriate task list and you immediately know all the things you need to do.

At home, similarly you may have separate lists for things you have to do around the house—for example, things that need repair, items you need to purchase at the mall, or things you have to do to prepare for a dinner party or a vacation.

Paper planners that are ring-bound (e.g., Filofax) allow for easy maintenance of separate tabbed lists at the back for each project/category. New sheets can be easily inserted as needed. Digital planners easily allow for set up of multiple (e.g., 15 or more) separate task lists.

3. Check off items in the paper planner or "delete/purge" in the digital planner as soon as they are completed (very satisfying!).

V. TIPS FOR SUCCESSFUL SCHEDULING

1. Schedule tasks that repeat for the same time each day (e.g., weekend bill paying, laundry, dishes): regular **structure works best!**
2. People who work freelance or from their homes should observe regular business hours for work-related tasks as much as possible, and defer the temptation to do errands, or recreate, until the evenings or weekends.
3. Plan to do the more difficult/challenging things when you will be most motivated (e.g., before/after a meeting when you're all fired up about the issue and the plans under consideration).
4. If you find that you have a lot of energy, do the most difficult thing first—that is, the thing you have been putting off the longest, or the thing you are not likely to have an opportunity to do again.
5. On the other hand, if you are tired, do that which is easiest, or that which is "automatic"—requires the least active thought or effort—or that which is the most fun/enjoyable.

6. Never leave off a task in the middle of a difficult part. It will be that much harder to pick it up again.

7. Schedule larger blocks of time for things that require a lot of mental "start up" (e.g., writing).

8. Fit little things in the "time cracks"—for example, while waiting in line or while in the car/bus/subway (see list below).

9. If you fall off the "horse" (i.e., the schedule), as you inevitably will do, don't spend time berating yourself. Just get right back up and get back on!

10. Be sure to schedule "downtime" (relaxation time). If you don't, you will come to feel that you "never have a moment's rest," and you will come to hate your schedule.

VI. Using the "Time Cracks" (a Few Things You Can Do While Waiting)

We all experience "downtime" during the day. These small "slices of time" can be put to good use (and save valuable time later). Examples of things that can be done during these "time cracks" are the following:

- Plan schedule.
- Address/stamp an envelope.
- Make a list.
- Decide on dinner, weekend, gift, what to wear to a party, what to do the next day at the office.
- Generate ideas for a project or paper.
- Listen to books on tape.
- Observe location of various stores and businesses along the road while in slow traffic.
- Have a good book or newspaper along with you.
- Do mental long-term planning. Set aside "sacred" time each week for this as well.

TAKE-HOME NOTES

Time Management
Time Awareness and Scheduling

REMEMBER: ***If it's not in the planner, it doesn't exist!***

I. INTRODUCTION

For many individuals with ADHD, time is a problem. When work needs to be done, there is not enough of it. When you have to wait for something, there is too much of it. For some, time seems like an enemy; for others, time is a mystery. But successfully using and managing time is essential to most careers and endeavors. Whether you're a student, mechanic, housewife, CEO, or surgeon, to succeed, you need to manage your time. When we talk about time management we are going to talk about the skills and tools you need to complete tasks as efficiently and quickly as you want or need to do them. Having a good awareness of time is the first step in good time management. Research has shown that people with ADHD are poor at estimating time. This means you may not be a good judge of how long certain tasks take. You may also be a poor judge of how much time has elapsed while you're engaged in a task. How can you change this?

II. IMPROVING YOUR TIME AWARENESS

This is a skill that requires practice, practice, practice. The exercise for this week, and for subsequent weeks throughout the program, will be to record the amount of time your daily activities take. This can be a slightly laborious process but it will also help you enormously in better managing your time. To plan effectively you need an accurate and reasonable idea of how much time it takes you to complete things.

(cont.)

III. MAKE THE CLOCK YOUR CONSTANT COMPANION

Good time management is impossible unless there is a clock or watch within view at all times. You are never able to say, "I didn't know what time it was," if there is a clock staring you in the face in every room. We run into trouble when we assume that we can estimate the passage of time accurately without actually consulting a clock. Test yourself sometime: Without looking at your watch, see if you can guess what time it is (e.g., by thinking back to what you have done since the last time you checked the time). With practice, you will find that you get better and better at estimating how much time has elapsed. If you are not focused on keeping track of time, it will slip away from you.

IV. "COMMANDMENTS" OF PLANNER USE

1. Thou may have one planner and one planner only. You must choose one planner; commit to it and stick with it.

2. Thou must carry thy planner with thee at all times. The planner must be portable and you must have it with you at all times to check appointment times, enter items to do, and so on. If you run into someone on the street and the opportunity arises to schedule an appointment, you want to have your planner available.

3. Thou shalt enter every appointment and task into thy planner! This is where one makes the commitment to completing the appointment or the task. Unless and until it is entered into the planner, it does not exist and therefore surely will not get done!

4. Thou shalt consult thy planner every morning, every midday, and every evening! (In other words, you may not start your day without a plan!) What's in the planner will have no impact on your life unless you consult it regularly—as regularly as you brush your teeth. It must become a thrice-daily habit. You consult it at night to make plans for the morning for travel, wardrobe, office materials, and so on that you need to bring the next day. You consult it in the morning to remind yourself of what is scheduled for the day so as to "hit the ground running" as the day begins and to ensure that nothing is forgotten. You need to consult it at midday to revise and reprioritize the activities for the afternoon, given the events of the morning. **At least once a day, you must update the planner, and reschedule the uncompleted items. Set a "cue" for yourself to remember to check your planner—for example, when you're making your coffee in the morning, during your lunch break, and when you're setting your alarm clock at night.**

V. SCHEDULING

Learning to schedule and use scheduling tools is really just a specialized form of being organized. We'll talk about some systems, but you will have to find what works for you. But you *must* have a system and *you must use it every day*.

(cont.)

Short-Term Scheduling

This means that:

- All appointments should be recorded.
- All tasks should be scheduled.
- All tasks that are not completed must be moved to the next time period.
- The schedule should be reviewed and updated daily—***Pick a time of day and do it at that time faithfully!***

Tips for Successful Scheduling

1. Schedule tasks that repeat for the same time each day (e.g., weekend bill paying, laundry, dishes). Regular **structure works best!**
2. People who work freelance or from their homes should observe regular business hours for work-related tasks as much as possible, and defer the temptation to do errands, or recreate, until the evenings or weekends.
3. Plan to do the more difficult/challenging things when you will be most motivated (e.g., before/after a meeting when you're all fired up about the issue and the plans under consideration).
4. If you find that you have a lot of energy, do the most difficult thing first—that is, the thing you have been putting off the longest, or the thing you are not likely to have an opportunity to do again.
5. On the other hand, if you are tired, do that which is easiest, or that which is "automatic"—requires the least active thought or effort—or that which is the most fun/enjoyable.
6. Never leave off a task in the middle of a difficult part. It will be that much harder to pick it up again.
7. Schedule larger blocks of time for things that require a lot of mental "start up" (e.g., writing).
8. Fit little things in the "time cracks"—for example, while waiting on a line or while in the car/bus/subway (see list below).
9. If you fall off the "horse" (i.e., the schedule), as you inevitably will do, don't spend time berating yourself. Just get right back up and get back on!
10. Be sure to schedule "downtime" (relaxation time). If you don't, you will come to feel that you "never have a moment's rest," and you will come to hate your schedule.

VI. USING THE "TIME CRACKS" (A FEW THINGS YOU CAN DO WHILE WAITING)

We all experience "downtime" during the day. These "slices of time" can be put to good use (and save valuable time later). Examples of things that can be done during these "time cracks" are the following:

(cont.)

- Plan schedule.
- Address/stamp an envelope.
- Make a list.
- Decide on dinner, weekend, gift, what to wear to a party, what to do the next day at the office.
- Generate ideas for a project or paper.
- Listen to books on tape.
- Observe location of various stores and businesses along the road while in slow traffic.
- Have a good book or newspaper along with you.
- Do mental long-term planning. Set aside "sacred" time each week for this as well.

TAKE-HOME EXERCISE

Time Management
Time Awareness and Scheduling

I. EVALUATE YOUR CURRENT PLANNER AND OBTAIN A NEW ONE (IF NECESSARY)

You may have only one planner—do not delay the decision.

Check in the space if your current planner has these **essential** features:

_____ 1. Easily portable—can be carried with you **every** day

_____ 2. Easy for **you** to use. If you are not comfortable with computers, then an electronic personal digital assistant (PDA) may not be best for you.

_____ 3. Has ample space for **daily** to-do lists and longer-term project lists.

_____ 4. Can be easily updated—that is, has sheets for the date book, address section, and to-do lists that can be removed and replaced (as in a Filofax).

Note: If your planner does not have these features, you must purchase a new one—before the next session!

II. INCREASING TIME AWARENESS

Next to each item below write down how much time you think it usually takes. Enter in the additional spaces in the left column some items from your own personal routine. When the next opportunity comes for each of these, actually time yourself on each of these items and record the actual time in the column on the right.

(cont.)

	Estimated time to complete	Start	Finish	Actual elapsed time
Getting ready for work	_____	_____	_____	_____
Commuting to work (school, store, etc.)	_____	_____	_____	_____
Preparing dinner	_____	_____	_____	_____
Sorting the mail	_____	_____	_____	_____
Going to the bank	_____	_____	_____	_____
Reading e-mail	_____	_____	_____	_____
Preparing a business letter	_____	_____	_____	_____
Paying bills	_____	_____	_____	_____
Returning daily phone calls	_____	_____	_____	_____
Emptying the dishwasher	_____	_____	_____	_____
Doing the dishes	_____	_____	_____	_____
Walking the dog	_____	_____	_____	_____
Exercising (include commute to gym if applicable)	_____	_____	_____	_____
_____	_____	_____	_____	_____
_____	_____	_____	_____	_____
_____	_____	_____	_____	_____

III. WHERE DOES THE TIME GO? MAKE A TIME LOG

It's hard to make changes in how we manage time, if we don't know where the time goes now. In order to answer this question, this exercise asks you to select a weekday and track everything you do—that is, make a log and fill in all of your activities. You may find it convenient to keep a running log in your planner and list times within hourly time slots, beginning with your wake-up, commute to work, arrival at work, and so on. If there is insufficient space, then make a copy of the calendar page before it is filled in. Or use the form on the next page. Then, you might fill it in like this:

9:00–10:00	Worked on memo
10:00–11:00	E-mail
11:00–Noon	Meeting
Noon–1:00	Lunch

You should have at least one entry for each hour, continuing through to bedtime.

(cont.)

DAILY ACTIVITY LOG

Date: _____

Time interval	Activity
5 A.M.–6 A.M.	
6 A.M.–7 A.M.	
7 A.M.–8 A.M.	
8 A.M.–9 A.M.	
9 A.M.–10 A.M.	
10 A.M.–11 A.M.	
11 A.M.–Noon	
Noon–1 P.M.	
1 P.M.–2 P.M.	
2 P.M.–3 P.M.	
3 P.M.–4 P.M.	
4 P.M.–5 P.M.	
5 P.M.–6 P.M.	
6 P.M.–7 P.M.	
7 P.M.–8 P.M.	
8 P.M.–9 P.M.	
9 P.M.–10 P.M.	
10 P.M.–11 P.M.	
11 P.M.–Midnight	
Midnight–1 A.M.	
1 A.M.–2 A.M.	
2 A.M.–3 A.M.	
3 A.M.–4 A.M.	
4 A.M.–5 A.M.	

LEADER NOTES

Time Management

Making Tasks Manageable and Rewarding Yourself

New Target Skills:

- Breaking down large or aversive tasks into manageable chunks.
- Contingent self-reinforcement.

In-Session Exercises:

- Break down complex or difficult task into parts.
- Generate a personal reward list.

Take-Home Exercise:

- Schedule and complete one or more small tasks (< 1 hour).
- Continue time-estimation and time-logging exercises as needed.

Today we're going to talk about using rewards to make unpleasant tasks more pleasant. Tasks that are repetitious, boring, tedious, or effortful are particularly difficult for people with ADHD. A very effective way to deal with these is to break them down into manageable "chunks," and to reward yourself after the completion of each "chunk."

REMEMBER: *If you're having trouble getting started,*
then the first step is too big!

This statement is inexorably and inevitably true. The implication is that you must continue to reduce the magnitude of what you intend to do (or the time you intend to spend) until you feel that you can **easily** accomplish it.

Example: If you are facing a mound of papers on your desk that you feel you can barely look at, much less organize, decide how many minutes you could easily tolerate spending on the task. Let's say you decide on an hour. Now 3 hours have gone by and you find you still haven't started on the task. Obviously, then, 60 minutes was still too long for you to plan to spend on the task. So then, you try a new agreement with yourself to spend 30 minutes. Still not starting? Then plan to do just 15 minutes. You might try setting a timer for the allotted time. *The idea is to keep reducing the number of minutes until you feel that it would be "no sweat" to work on it for that long and you actually start on the task.* When you finish the allotted number of minutes, certainly feel free to keep on going if you are "into" it (as you may well be)! *If not, schedule yourself for the next period of time (at least the same number of minutes) when you will work on it again.*

Other examples: Say you have to repair a leak or do another home repair task that you don't enjoy and have been avoiding. A helpful approach here might be to make the first step to just assemble the materials needed to complete the task and put them into some obvious place. Similarly, if you have to assemble a piece of furniture or an appliance, just read the instructions first and see what is involved. If you have to write a business letter, collect the files/documents you will need. This will serve two functions—it will get you started on the task and it will create a visual cue that will remind you to complete the task.

Folks with ADHD are better "sprinters" than long-distance runners. Therefore, you should set up/manage time accordingly—that is, plan to do only a small amount at one time.

Other ways to use rewards are the following:

1. *Plan to give yourself a reward ("reinforcer") after completing a task or part of a task that is difficult or unpleasant ("contingent self-reward").* Such self-rewards may include taking a walk, calling a friend, surfing the Net, reading a book or magazine, watching one show on TV, listening to music, fixing a snack, exercising, taking a hot bath, or any of a host of individually preferred items. If you find you are having difficulty starting or completing the task, think of the reward you will be able to have as soon as you are finished.

2. *Use naturally occurring reinforcers.* For example, if your business responsibilities involve writing memos and making calls to colleagues and you enjoy talking to people much more than writing, write your memo first, and *then* allow yourself to make your call. Similarly, alternate the naturally more difficult and easier tasks or boring/interesting tasks throughout the day.

3. *Pair aversive tasks with pleasurable ones.* Some tasks or activities can be made more tolerable if they are *paired with* (*i.e., done at the same time as*) more pleasurable events or conditions. **Examples** include exercising while watching TV, a video, or listening to music; curling up in a comfortable chair to read a business document; housecleaning to lively music; and loading dishes in the dishwasher or cleaning counters while chatting on the phone with a friend. You may also consider using an efficient software program to accomplish a difficult task (e.g., doing bill paying online, or using TurboTax to do your taxes).

4. *Partner with someone to do the task.* Either have someone stand by you while working on an unpleasant task or work on the task together.

IN-SESSION EXERCISE 1: BREAKING DOWN A LARGE TASK INTO MANAGEABLE "CHUNKS"

Ask the group for an example of a personal or business project that they have had trouble getting started on or completing. If no one volunteers anything, provide an example (e.g., cleaning or doing repairs on an entire house). Illustrate how one breaks the task into parts (e.g., by task—dusting, vacuuming, plastering; or by area—bathroom, roof), puts them onto a schedule, and plans a contingent self-reward after the completion of each.

IN-SESSION EXERCISE 2: GENERATING A PERSONAL REWARD LIST

Give each group member a sheet of paper and ask him or her to list small personal rewards (requiring 30 minutes or less) and larger rewards (1 or 2 hours).

> **NOTE TO THERAPIST:** Glance over to see how much each participant is writing. Inability to identify any rewarding activities is often a sign that the person is depressed.

CONTINUE TIME-RELATED EXERCISES AT HOME

Continue Time-Estimation Exercises

Stress that for those who want to increase their time-estimation abilities, continued practice in time estimation will be helpful. Pass out additional copies of the time-estimation exercise to be continued at home.

Continue Time-Logging Exercises

Continuing the time-logging exercise will help participants to gain a clearer picture of how time is spent and to monitor the success of planned changes in time allocations.

TAKE-HOME NOTES

Time Management
Making Tasks Manageable and Rewarding Yourself

REMEMBER: *If you're having trouble getting started, then the first step is too big!*

Tasks that are repetitious, boring, tedious, or effortful are particularly difficult for people with ADHD. A very effective way to deal with these is to break them down into manageable "chunks," and to reward yourself after the completion of each "chunk."

Example: Say you have to repair a leak or do another home repair task that you don't enjoy and have been avoiding. A helpful approach here might be to make the first step to just assemble the materials needed to complete the task and put them into some obvious place. This will serve two functions—it will get you started on the task and it will create a visual cue that will remind you to complete the task.

1. *Plan to give yourself a reward after completing a task or part of a task that is difficult or unpleasant.* Such self-rewards may include taking a walk, calling a friend, surfing the Net, reading a book or magazine, watching one show on TV, listening to music, fixing a snack, exercising, taking a hot bath, or any of a host of individually preferred items. If you find you are having difficulty starting or completing the task, think of the reward you will be able to have as soon as you are finished.

2. *Use naturally occurring reinforcers.* For example, if your business responsibilities involve writing memos and making calls to colleagues and you enjoy talking to people much more than writing, write your memo first, and *then* allow yourself to make your call. Similarly, alternate the naturally more difficult and easier tasks or boring/interesting tasks throughout the day.

(cont.)

---

3. *Pair aversive tasks with pleasurable ones.* Some tasks or activities can be made more tolerable if they are *paired with* (*i.e., done at the same time as*) more pleasurable events or conditions. **Examples** include exercising while watching TV, a video, or listening to music; curling up in a comfortable chair to read a business document; housecleaning to lively music; and loading dishes in the dishwasher or cleaning counters while chatting on the phone with a friend. You might also consider using an efficient software program to accomplish a difficult task (e.g., doing bill paying online, or using TurboTax to do your taxes).

4. *Partner with someone to do the task.* Either have someone stand by you while you work on an unpleasant task or work on the task together.

TAKE-HOME EXERCISE

Time Management
*Making Tasks Manageable
and Rewarding Yourself*

Step 1: Select one task you've been postponing/avoiding/procrastinating about. Select one that is simple and would easily take less than an hour to complete.

Step 2: Estimate (in minutes) how long the task will take and schedule it appropriately in your planner.

Step 3: Plan a pleasurable little reward to give yourself after completing the task.

Step 4: Time yourself, complete the task, and reward yourself appropriately.

Step 5: Complete the form on the next page.

If it went well, repeat all the steps for a second task that you have been putting off. If it didn't go well, write down in the log what went wrong—and try again!

Remember to continue time-estimation and time-logging exercises! With practice, your time-management skills will improve.

(cont.)

TIME LOG

Task selected	Estimated time to accomplish	Scheduled day and time	Completed?	Actual time needed
Task 1				
Task 2				

How did it go? Any problems?

Task 1

_____

_____

_____

_____

_____

_____

Task 2

_____

_____

_____

_____

_____

_____

(cont.)

TIME-ESTIMATION WORKSHEET

Developing the skill of time estimation requires continued practice. In order to get good at it, choose the tasks or activities that you want to become more punctual with and time yourself. On the blank lines add in those tasks/activities that are particularly concerning to you. (Make additional copies as needed.)

	Estimated time to complete	Start	Finish	Actual elapsed time
Getting ready for work				
Commuting to work (school, store, etc.)				
Preparing dinner				
Sorting the mail				
Going to the bank				
Reading e-mail				
Preparing a business letter				
Paying bills				
Returning daily phone calls				
Emptying the dishwasher				
Doing the dishes				
Walking the dog				
Exercising (include commute to gym, if applicable)				

(cont.)

DAILY ACTIVITY LOG

Date: _____

Time interval	Activity
5 A.M.–6 A.M.	
6 A.M.–7 A.M.	
7 A.M.–8 A.M.	
8 A.M.–9 A.M.	
9 A.M.–10 A.M.	
10 A.M.–11 A.M.	
11 A.M.–Noon	
Noon–1 P.M.	
1 P.M.–2 P.M.	
2 P.M.–3 P.M.	
3 P.M.–4 P.M.	
4 P.M.–5 P.M.	
5 P.M.–6 P.M.	
6 P.M.–7 P.M.	
7 P.M.–8 P.M.	
8 P.M.–9 P.M.	
9 P.M.–10 P.M.	
10 P.M.–11 P.M.	
11 P.M.–Midnight	
Midnight–1 A.M.	
1 A.M.–2 A.M.	
2 A.M.–3 A.M.	
3 A.M.–4 A.M.	
4 A.M.–5 A.M.	

Time Management

Prioritizing and To-Do Lists

New Target Skills:
- Identifying priorities.
- Use of planner for prioritizing.

In-Session Exercise:
- Transfer items from to-do list to schedule.

Take-Home Exercise:
- Complete importance–urgency grid.
- Schedule a week's to-do items.

REMEMBER: *Do all things in the order of priority!*

NOTE TO THERAPIST: Before reviewing the Take-Home Exercise, take a few minutes to review and highlight the following material (from the last session) with the group:

"Principles" of Scheduling

1. Estimate how long the task will take. (If the task is large, break it down into parts.)
2. Enter task into planner, being sure to allow sufficient time.
3. Plan (and allow time for) self-reinforcement (reward) afterward.

I. WHY PRIORITIZING IS IMPORTANT

- **There is simply not enough time to get everything done.** It is a truism that there simply aren't enough hours in the day to accomplish all that we would like to. Most of us, with or without ADHD, never get to all the items on our to-do lists. Therefore, it is essential that the most important things get done first!

- **Without prioritizing, people with ADHD will respond in the moment.** *Prioritizing is especially important for people with ADHD* who may be very prone to shift their attention to whatever is most stimulating or pressing at the moment. You will need to *actively* suppress that urge—and here it helps if you have *already committed* yourself to certain priority items, which you have *clearly* in mind.

II. HOW TO DECIDE ON PRIORITIES

Several things must be taken into account in deciding what should be done first.

Urgency/Deadlines

Those things that have the soonest deadline. *Ask yourself, as you look at your calendar, when does this have to be done?*

Importance

If you only attended to things that are urgent, you would always find yourself "putting out fires" (which, in fact, is a common experience of people with ADHD!). *The key here is to consider what is most important to one's own short- and long-term goals.*

So, for example, it may be more important to your job performance and job evaluation to do the tasks that directly increase sales (e.g., making cold calls to potential clients), rather than to spend that time on "in-house" projects.

Personal Goals, Values, and Objectives

Your personal **long-term goals** and values must be considered. So, for example, if your long-term goal is to be a writer or composer, and working in a business is just your "day job," you may want to prioritize your daily work so that you give your best hour(s) early in the morning or at another time of day to your creative project, and give only what is necessary to your desk job. The same is true for any project that will reap rewards only in the long term.

Relationships: If an important value is the amount of time spent with your family or friends, you may want to make it a priority to be home with them at a certain time in the evening or preserve certain hours to spend with them on the weekend.

Exercise is another example of a personal goal that has very great long-term importance but relatively little short-term importance and no urgency whatever. Unless you prioritize this activity in your daily schedule based on its long-term importance for your health, it is unlikely that you will ever get to it. In fact, this is true of many activities that are important to our long-term well-being.

Efficiency and Feasibility

There are more and less efficient ways to plan one's time and organize daily activities. One rule of thumb is to ***group like things together***. For example, if you have phone calls to make, it may be a good idea to group them together on your planner task list, and do them all at once. Similarly, if you have shopping and other errands to do, plan to go to all the stores that are close to each other on the same excursion, rather than making a special trip out of your way for one item.

Plan your time so as to ***make use of the "time cracks"*** (Session 2). A simple example: If you are making pasta and you know that you can't do anything with the pasta until the water is boiling, put the water on the stove first thing, and do another step (e.g., make the salad) while you wait for the water to boil.

If You Still Can't Decide What to Do First . . .

Another way to determine your priorities is to simply ask yourself, ***"What will I feel good about accomplishing today?"***

Priorities will change in the course of a day . . . depending on how much you get done and new tasks, issues, and problems that arise. In the middle of the day when you review your planner, it's a good idea to review your task list simultaneously for any adjustments that need to be made to your priorities for the remainder of the day.

NOTE TO THERAPIST: People with ADHD frequently voice **two sources of reluctance** or resistance to scheduling tasks and other activities in their planners. One source is the desire to preserve large swaths of time during which they have the freedom "to do anything." It is important to help participants recognize that the opportunity to "do anything" here is really an illusion and that not planning anything will more often usually mean that *nothing* will get done. Once again it is the case that "If it's not in the planner, it doesn't exist." A second source of reluctance is the fear that noting tasks to complete in the planner for a given day/time will have the result of arousing feelings of failure and demoralization when, at the end of the day, they must confront the evidence that, once again, they did not complete the items on their to-do list. The therapist can be supportive here by highlighting that the participant is acquiring new tools that will help him or her be more successful in completing those items—and, toward that end, it will be helpful to review how the time was spent, whether too many items were scheduled, and so on.

IN-SESSION EXERCISE: PRIORITIZING AND SCHEDULING

   1. Ask for someone to volunteer the items on his or her to-do list. Make a weeklong calendar on the board with columns for each of the 7 days and three rows for morning, afternoon, and evening time blocks. With the input of the group, transfer the items on the to-do list to their appropriate places on the weekly calendar, applying insofar as possible all the principles of scheduling discussed previously, including time estimation, breaking down complex or aversive tasks into parts, and following each with a reinforcer, as well as the new material from this session.

   2. If no one volunteers, work with the following or a similar list of items. Begin by scheduling for a single day with "spillover" as necessary for subsequent days.

> 11:00 A.M. meeting with boss.
> Lunch with colleague.
> 4:00 P.M. deadline for material to printer.
> Proofread copy before it goes to printer.
> Mail letters.
> 1:30 P.M. phone conference with child's teacher.
> Buy milk.
> Prepare agenda for 11:00 A.M. meeting with boss.
> Review day's schedule (twice).
> 8:00 P.M. dinner for friend's birthday.

Buy birthday card.
Order theater tickets.
Complete budget for next Tuesday's meeting.
Call Client A.
Call Client B.
Work up business plan for new project.

IMPORTANCE–URGENCY GRID

One way to think about priorities is to use the following grid, taken from Stephen Covey's (1989) highly successful book, The Seven Habits of Highly Effective People*

	Urgent	Not urgent
Important	I—Important and urgent	II—Important but not urgent
Not important	III—Not important but urgent	IV—Not important and not urgent

I—Important and Urgent

These are the things that have the highest priority. For example: Your child is sick and you have to stay home from work. You have to prepare a report for the boss that has a firm deadline. You have to submit your graduate school applications by the deadline. You have to prepare for a final exam, or a licensing or qualifying test. These are clearly of major importance and can't be put off.

II—Important but Not Urgent

These are generally items, such as attending to our important personal goals or nurturing our relationships that, as we have described, relate to our long-term career success, or our personal well-being and development. Although they may be extremely important in determining our long-term personal satisfaction in life, their lack of urgency on a day-to-day basis means that they are the most likely to be neglected, shunted aside, or overwhelmed by the daily demands of items in Quadrants I and III.

---

*Reprinted with permission from Franklin Covey Co.

III—Not Important but Urgent

Without a conscious effort to do otherwise, it is possible to spend the majority of one's day on these items. There is a particular risk for people with ADHD here in that these are the demands that impinge most on our daily consciousness as they are the most salient and obvious—phone calls, interruptions, e-mails, and so on. Some of these may be important, but more often they are things that *other* people need urgently—for example, the paperwork that has to be completed and returned by a deadline, or the meeting this afternoon that all staff must attend. You may feel and look "busy" while doing these things, but you may not necessarily be accomplishing anything much.

Note that unless we actively plan to do otherwise—to complete tasks and projects *before* their due date—urgent items can easily come to constitute the totality of what we do every day. We will be constantly putting out fires!

IV—Not Important and Not Urgent

These are the things that deservedly have the lowest priority. At the office, some of these things may simply be time wasters. At home, they may be the things that "it would be nice to do someday" (e.g., redecorate the bedroom). Because they are often appealing projects or pleasant activities, there is a great risk that people with ADHD will devote time and attention to these items, neglecting the more important and urgent ones. In that case, consider scheduling these as recreational activities for "downtime." Other items in this category may be tasks that could easily be delegated to others. Alternatively, these may be items that should be reevaluated and deleted from one's priority list altogether!

TAKE-HOME NOTES

Time Management
Prioritizing and To-Do Lists

REMEMBER: *Do all things in the order of priority!*

CREATING AND PRIORITIZING TO-DO LISTS

In addition to appointments, it is crucial to:

- Have daily and weekly to-do lists.
- Prioritize your list.

Organization experts suggest that you should have a place where you write down **everything** that you need to do, regardless of how urgent. This ensures that it won't be forgotten. But if you left it at that, you'd have a page full of things to do, with no plan or organization of how to do them. This master list should be reviewed daily. Next to each item should be a ranking (hot, warm, cold or 1, 2, 3, etc.) to show the item's priority or urgency. From this master list a daily or weekly to-do list is generated, taking those items with the highest priority. These are then scheduled in your planner.

In summary, you must:

- Sort tasks by priority and similarity (it takes less time to do similar tasks together, because you have all the equipment you need—e.g., make all phone calls at the same time, type correspondence, pay several bills rather than just one).
- Use a priority system such as "hot, warm, cold"; "now, soon, later"; or "A, B, C"—whatever works for you.

(cont.)

---

10 TAKE-HOME TIPS

1. Estimate how much time will be needed and allocate time in the schedule accordingly.

2. Schedule larger, uninterrupted blocks of time for things that require more focus and concentration. Once you get going on something you may want to be able to devote more time to it. Take advantage of natural momentum in planning your time.

3. For greatest efficiency, schedule similar things together (e.g., plan out your errand route so that you go to the places nearest each other at the same time).

4. Consider your internal clock—schedule the more difficult, demanding things for the times when you are freshest and most alert.

5. Schedule the easier, more enjoyable things (e.g., phone calls, e-mails) as a reward *after* you have completed something more difficult/demanding. Alternate the harder tasks with the easier ones.

6. When possible, pair aversive tasks with pleasurable activities.

   Exercise while watching TV.

   Load the dishwasher while talking on the phone.

   Put lively music on while housecleaning.

7. Limit social and other nonwork, and home errands/tasks to nonbusiness hours (e.g., after 5 P.M. and on weekends).

8. Always *prioritize* the tasks of the day and review your priority list first thing before you start out in the morning. Try with all your might to resist the temptation to do things out of priority order. Priority should depend upon the following:

   Urgency/deadline.

   Importance.

   Long-term goals and values.

   Efficiency and feasibility.

9. Always carry your planner with you.

10. And remember:

REMEMBER: ***If you're having trouble getting started, then the first step is too big***
(i.e., break down the task into smaller, more manageable parts).

TAKE-HOME EXERCISE

Time Management

Prioritizing and To-Do Lists

TAKE-HOME EXERCISE, PART I

Use the following exercise to get a better sense of whether your current energy and time allocations are truly in sync with your long-term goals and values.

Step 1. Using the grid on the next page, as discussed in the session, write down the main types of tasks/projects/activities and so on that currently fall into each category for *you*.

Step 2. Estimate what percent of your total time is spent in the activities in each quadrant.

Step 3. Do you think that the percent allocations for each quadrant reflect their importance in your job and in your life? If not, how can you pull time from any of the other quadrants into Quadrant II, which has the items most important for your long-term personal success and satisfaction? Indicate the changes below and/or make these changes to the grid by using a different color pen or pencil to cross out or "drag" items (via arrows) to different quadrants.

_____

_____

_____

_____

(cont.)

	Urgent	Not Urgent
Important	**I—Important and urgent**	**II—Important but not urgent**
	Estimated percent _____	Estimated percent _____
Not important	**III—Not important but urgent**	**IV—Not important and not urgent**
	Estimated percent _____	Estimated percent _____

Grid reprinted with permission from Franklin Covey Co.

(cont.)

TAKE-HOME EXERCISE, PART II

Use the form on the next page for this exercise.

Step 1: Make a list of those tasks/activities you would like to accomplish **in the coming week**. In particular, identify those things that you have been putting off or that you are unlikely to accomplish unless you make a special effort. If you are having trouble prioritizing, ask yourself, "What will I feel really good about having accomplished today?"

List these items on the next page in column 1. It's best to start with a modest list—for example, not more than 6 to 10 items.

Step 2: If there is a deadline or a particular day on which the item must be accomplished, indicate that in Column 2.

Step 3: Estimate how long the task or activity will take. Indicate this in Column 3.

Step 4: Assign each item a priority score from 1 to 5, in which "1" has the highest priority score and "5" the lowest. Indicate this in Column 4.

Step 5: *Schedule for a specific day and time and transfer each item to the appropriate day and time in your planner.*

Step 6: Indicate on the form when you accomplish each item.

(cont.)

A WEEK'S TO-DO LIST

Task/activity to do	Date/ deadline	Estimated time needed	Priority (1 to 5)	Scheduled for (day and time)	Date completed

LEADER NOTES

Time Management
Overcoming Emotional Obstacles

New Target Skills:
- Identifying automatic thoughts.
- Labeling cognitive distortions.
- Defusing distressing feelings by challenging and revising automatic thoughts.

In-Session Exercise:
- Identify and revise cognitive distortions.

Take-Home Exercise:
- Identify and correct automatic thoughts (with sample).

NOTE TO THERAPIST: To allow additional time for assimilation of the material in this session, it may be broken into two sessions: Use the first to discuss *identifying* the cognitive distortions (i.e., the material in outline sections A, B, and C below), and the second to discuss *challenging* those thoughts (material in sections D and E). The Take-Home Exercise would be divided accordingly—that is, up to item 4 for the first Take-Home Exercise, and items 5 through 7 for the second session.

I. How Emotions Affect Efficiency

1. People with ADHD often procrastinate or avoid certain tasks out of **depression or anxiety**. They have a history of failing when they have attempted to accomplish certain things, and they fear that their performance will be inadequate again.

- Depression may be reflected in demoralization and hopelessness that any effort will pay off—therefore, the feeling may be "Why even try?"
- Anxiety may be associated with fear of failure, which may lead a person to avoid certain tasks that are anticipated to be difficult or challenging to complete. An unrealistic **need for perfection** or for **total control or certainty of the outcome** may also inhibit him or her from getting started.

2. Children with ADHD are often **resistant or oppositional** to the demands, instructions, or expectations of others—particularly those "in authority." Unfortunately, this attitude may persist into adulthood when the effect of resisting may self-sabotage the goals and best interests of the person him- or herself.

Today we will focus on the understanding and treatment of anxiety and depression, as they may exacerbate ADHD symptoms. Next time we will talk about "oppositionality."

II. COGNITIVE-BEHAVIORAL THERAPY

A. *The Cognitive-Behavioral Model*

Cognitive therapy, which was developed by Aaron T. Beck, is based on the cognitive model. The basic premise of the cognitive model is that one's emotions and behaviors are influenced by **ways of thinking** about events and experiences. The following is based on the description of the model by Judith Beck (1995).

One's perception of the situation generates the feelings. Often however, the thoughts are so quick and automatic we are only aware of the feelings that follow.

With practice, we can become more aware of these thoughts, referred to as **automatic thoughts**.

NOTE TO THERAPIST: Make diagram on board to illustrate as you go.

Event → Automatic Thought → Reaction (Emotion, Behavior,
                                              and/or Physiological Reaction)

Automatic thoughts are quick evaluations of events. Sometimes they are accurate and at other times they are not.

Example ("John" writing article)

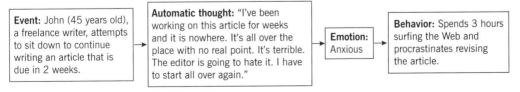

Event: John (45 years old), a freelance writer, attempts to sit down to continue writing an article that is due in 2 weeks.

Automatic thought: "I've been working on this article for weeks and it is nowhere. It's all over the place with no real point. It's terrible. The editor is going to hate it. I have to start all over again."

Emotion: Anxious

Behavior: Spends 3 hours surfing the Web and procrastinates revising the article.

B. How Do You Know When You're Having an Automatic Thought?

To better manage the feelings of anxiety and depression one must first become an observer and begin to identify the automatic thoughts that trigger these feelings and behaviors (e.g., avoidance or perfectionism).

The first step is to take note when you experience a change in feeling that is distressing. Label the feeling and pose the questions "What went through my mind at that point in time?" "What were the words or images?"

Example: Say you had an assignment for work or school due tomorrow and you plan to be up most of the night to complete it. As you sit down to work, you might have a sudden intense negative feeling, you may even have a feeling right now, as you imagine it. The first step is to think "What went through my head just then?" We are working backward from the feeling to the thought because the feelings are generally more salient.

The automatic thoughts are always directly related to the **type** of feeling in some way.

1. If the feeling is **anxiety**, the thought might be "Oh darn, what if I lose my job. I'll have to borrow more money. I won't be able to afford this apartment."
2. If the feeling is **depression**, an example of an automatic thought is "I don't really understand what I need to do. Why am I such an idiot?"
3. Finally, if the feeling is **anger**, the thought may be "How could my boss expect me to get this done in such a short period of time? He is so demanding. He wants me to fail."

C. "Bad" Automatic Thoughts: The "Cognitive Distortions"

NOTE TO THERAPIST: Ask the group members to turn to this page—the second page of their Take-Home Notes—as you review it with them.

• **All-or-nothing thinking** (may also be called perfectionism): Things are seen in black-or-white categories. For example: "If I don't get an 'A' on this, I'll be a total failure."

• **Overgeneralization:** A single negative event is seen as part of a comprehensive and interminable pattern. For example: "Everything in my life is a mess and will never get better"; "I never do anything right."

• **Selective attention:** A single negative detail is isolated and dwelt on exclusively. For example: "My boss hated my report" (when, in fact, he said that it was good overall but the conclusion needed editing).

- **Disqualifying the positives (closely related to selective attention):** Positive experiences are overlooked as "not counting," allowing the person to maintain a negative belief that is contradicted by everyday experiences. For example: Your friend says you look good in the outfit you're wearing, but you think you really look awful and that she's just saying it to be nice.

- **Jumping to conclusions:** Making a negative interpretation despite the absence of definite facts to support the conclusion. Two types:
  - **Mind reading:** Believing that someone is reacting negatively to oneself, without knowing for sure or checking it out with the other person. For example: You assume someone asks you for more information because he or she doubts the truth of what you are saying.
  - **Fortune-teller error:** Anticipating that things will turn out badly, and regarding the prediction as an already established fact. For example: "I *know* I'll make a fool of myself at the party and have a bad time—so I'd better not go."

- **Personalization:** Seeing oneself as the cause of some negative external event for which one is not, in fact, primarily responsible. For example: "That person must have left the room while I was speaking because I am so boring."

- **"Should" statements:** Maintaining excessive "shoulds," "musts," and "oughts" imply the need for guilt and punishment when unfulfilled. For example: "I *should* be able to work at top efficiency the entire day."

- **"Catastrophizing":** Believing that it would be a catastrophe if . . . a particular thing happened or didn't happen. For example: "It would be a catastrophe if I don't get this job and I couldn't stand it."

D. How to Get Rid of "Bad" Automatic Thoughts

Once we are able to identify the distortions in our automatic thoughts we want to **challenge** the distortion with a rational counterargument. For example, anxiety results in difficulties making decisions for fear of possible negative consequences of any course of action. In order to get past the inhibiting automatic thoughts it is necessary to substitute more positive thoughts.

In-Session Exercise: Examples of Automatic Thoughts, Cognitive Distortions, and Rational Responses

NOTE TO THERAPIST: For each item below, read and write the irrational belief and then ask the group to state:

1. What is the relevant cognitive distortion?
2. What is a more adaptive rational response?

1. **Situation:** The boss has just asked you to take on an important project.
   - **Automatic thought:** "I will fail at this, I always fail, so it would be better if I don't take it on at all."
   - **Cognitive distortions:** Overgeneralization, fortune-telling.
   - **Rational response:** "This is going to be a challenge, but I have succeeded at some challenges like this before. Even if I don't do perfectly well, I know I can at least do a decent job. It will show some of my skills and I will learn from the experience. My boss wouldn't have asked me to do it if he didn't think I could."

2. **Situation:** You get a call from a friend asking whether you have finished your share of a project you're working on together (and you haven't).
   - **Automatic thought:** "I can't finish anything. I guess I'm really just a lazy person."
   - **Cognitive distortion:** Overgeneralization.
   - **Rational response:** "I do have difficulty with follow-through but that doesn't mean I'm lazy. If I work for an hour at a time and allow myself a reward after each hour, I will be closer to finishing."

3. **Situation:** You get a "C" or "average" rating on a test or other form of evaluation.
   - **Automatic thought:** "I guess I'm really not very smart at all. I'm never going to be a success in college/graduate school/at this job."
   - **Cognitive distortions:** All-or-nothing thinking, fortune-telling.
   - **Rational response:** "There are many things I can do well. I don't have to be able to be do everything perfectly. Doing well or doing my personal best is enough. **'The Perfect is the enemy of the Good.'**"

4. **Situation:** You just complete something you've been putting off for months.
   - **Automatic thought:** "Well—I should have been able to do that a long time ago. I still haven't gotten around to taking care of X, Y, or Z. . . ."
   - **Cognitive distortion:** Disqualifying the positives—often indicative of depression. These thoughts are self-sabotaging because the person never takes credit for his or her successes. Even after he or she makes some progress, he or she devalues it. Tragically, it often means that the person stays demoralized and "stuck" and loses motivation to continue to work.
   - **Rational response:** "I did finish it. Given how difficult that usually is for me, that's a real step forward. Now maybe I can take on something else."

5. **Situation:** The night before a job interview.
   - **Automatic thought:** "I'm really worried about how well I'm going to do in this interview. I always get nervous in these situations and I **never** present myself in the best light. It would be just *awful* if I blow it—I'll never find another job like this one—or maybe this will always happen to me and I'll never get another job at all."

- **Cognitive distortions**: Catastrophizing, overgeneralizing, fortune-telling.
- **Rational response**: "So I may get a little nervous, but everybody is a little nervous in this situation; the interviewer knows that. I have a very good résumé and that will also show what I can do. I'll rehearse some answers to possible questions, and then I'll feel more confident going in."

E. *Where Do These Automatic Thoughts Come From?*

Adults with ADHD may be particularly vulnerable to feelings of anxiety and depression because of **core beliefs** about themselves as "incompetent," "stupid," and "not good enough." These beliefs often develop as a result of being criticized and demoralized in childhood for unintentional "mistakes."

> **NOTE TO THERAPIST:** As you speak, add the boxes for the "Core Belief" and then the "Relevant Childhood Data" to the diagram for "John" already on the board. Add an arrow to direct these to "Automatic Thought" in the diagram, as shown below.

Relevant Childhood Data

John has ADHD and an LD in math.
Now a freelance writer.

Father:
A successful businessman.
Demanded an orderly and efficient household.
Alcoholic, emotionally abusive toward John and his mother, often calling them "stupid."

Mother:
Scattered and easily overwhelmed.

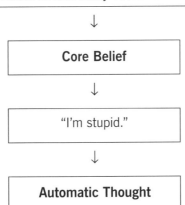

↓

Core Belief

↓

"I'm stupid."

↓

Automatic Thought

The result: So . . . thoughts about not being "good enough," or even "failing," may create anxiety and hold the individual back from trying new things, learning new skills (including organizational skills!), or undertaking new endeavors. In this example, John procrastinates instead of making further headway on the article.

The person may overcompensate and set his or her sights on unachievable "perfection" or self-reliance. In this example, John may obsess over every word and never feel he has gotten it "right."

TAKE-HOME NOTES

Time Management
Overcoming Emotional Obstacles

I. DEALING WITH EMOTIONAL DISTRACTERS

Cognitive theory suggests that distorted thoughts generate feelings of depression and anxiety and ineffective behaviors. Such thoughts are referred to as **automatic thoughts**. The thoughts are often so immediate we don't even notice them.

Individuals with ADHD may be at greater risk for anxiety and depression because their automatic thoughts become **distorted** over time as a result of perceived "mistakes" or "failures." Such moods may perpetuate the difficulties individuals already have with getting started on a task or they can produce internal distraction during a task or project, and keep you from following through. You may, for example, negatively evaluate your performance as you go along, decide it is not good enough, become depressed, and give up prematurely. You may think that if you aren't doing "perfectly" or if you get off your schedule, that "all is lost."

The **first step** in managing and changing feelings of depression and anxiety is to become aware of the automatic thoughts that trigger these feelings. Begin to take note of when you feel anxiety or depression. Try to label the feelings (e.g., anxiety, depression, anger, shame) and then ask yourself, "What went through my head just then? What were the words or images?" Some of the automatic thoughts are very likely to be **cognitive distortions**. Refer to the list on the next page.

The **second step** toward change is to challenge the distorted automatic thoughts and provide an alternative script. The following questions (Beck, 1995) will assist you in challenging the cognitive distortions:

- What is the evidence that the automatic thought is true?
- What is the evidence that the automatic thought is *not* true?
- Is there an alternative explanation?
- What's the worst that can happen?
- Could I live through it?

(cont.)

- What is the best that could happen?
- What is the most realistic outcome?
- What's the effect of my believing the automatic thought?
- What could be the effect of changing my thinking?
- What should I do about it?
- What would I tell a friend if he or she were in the same situation?

II. THE COGNITIVE DISTORTIONS

- **All-or-nothing thinking** (may also be called perfectionism): Things are seen in black-or-white categories. For example: "If I don't get an 'A' on this, I'll be a total failure."

- **Overgeneralization:** A single negative event is seen as part of a comprehensive and interminable pattern. For example: "Everything in my life is a mess and will never get better"; "I never do anything right."

- **Selective attention:** A single negative detail is isolated and dwelt on exclusively. For example: "My boss hated my report" (when, in fact, he said that it was good overall but the conclusion needed editing).

- **Disqualifying the positives (closely related to selective attention):** Positive experiences are overlooked as "not counting," allowing the person to maintain a negative belief that is contradicted by everyday experiences. For example: Your friend says you look good in the outfit you're wearing, but you think you really look awful and that she's just saying it to be nice.

- **Jumping to conclusions:** Making a negative interpretation despite the absence of definite facts to support the conclusion. Two types:
    - **Mind reading:** Believing that someone is reacting negatively to oneself, without knowing for sure or checking it out with the other person. For example: You assume someone asks you for more information because he or she doubts the truth of what you are saying.
    - **Fortune-teller error:** Anticipating that things will turn out badly, and regarding the prediction as an already established fact. For example: "I *know* I'll make a fool of myself at the party and have a bad time—so I'd better not go."

- **Personalization:** Seeing oneself as the cause of some negative external event for which one is not, in fact, primarily responsible. For example: "That person must have left the room while I was speaking because I am so boring."

- **"Should" statements:** Maintaining excessive "shoulds," "musts," and "oughts" imply the need for guilt and punishment when unfulfilled. For example: "I *should* be able to work at top efficiency the entire day."

- **"Catastrophizing":** Believing that it would be a catastrophe if . . . a particular thing happened or didn't happen. For example: "It would be a catastrophe if I don't get this job and I couldn't stand it."

TAKE-HOME EXERCISE

Time Management
Overcoming Emotional Obstacles

IDENTIFYING AND CHALLENGING AUTOMATIC THOUGHTS

The next time you find yourself procrastinating or feeling anxious or depressed about getting started on a task, activity, or chore, complete the following. It's best to do it as you're trying to start—while you're still in the situation—or as soon as possible thereafter so you don't forget important details.

1. **How are you feeling? (anxious, depressed, guilty, angry, etc.)**

   _____

   _____

2. **What is the current situation, event, task, or activity that you are faced with? What are you currently doing in the situation? (For example, responding to distractions—e.g., Internet, magazines, TV, pacing around.) Be as descriptive as possible.**

   _____

   _____

   _____

3. **Write down all the thoughts you are having in the situation—tune in particularly to thoughts you are having about *yourself*.**

   _____

   _____

   _____

   _____

   _____

(cont.)

4. **Now, look back at your automatic thoughts. What cognitive distortions do you recognize there? (Refer to your thoughts in 3. and write out all those that apply.)**

_____ All-or-nothing thinking _____

_____ Overgeneralization _____

_____ Selective attention _____

_____ Disqualifying the positives _____

_____ Personalization _____

_____ "Should" statements _____

_____ Catastrophizing _____

Jumping to conclusions:

_____ Mind reading _____

_____ Fortune-teller error _____

5. **Challenge these negative thoughts (distortions) by responding to the following questions that apply.**

What is the evidence that the automatic thought is true?

_____

What is the evidence that the automatic thought is *not* true?

_____

Is there an alternative explanation?

_____

What's the worst that can happen?

_____

Could I live through it?

_____

What is the best that could happen?

_____

What is the most realistic outcome?

_____

(cont.)

What is the effect of my believing the automatic thought?

_____

What could be the effect of changing my thinking?

_____

What should I do about it?

_____

What would I tell a friend if he or she were in the same situation?

_____

6. **What are more rational thoughts in response to the situation?**

_____

_____

7. **Outcome—How do you feel now? How did the situation end?**

_____

_____

(cont.)

Sample of Completed Take-Home Exercise

IDENTIFYING AND CORRECTING AUTOMATIC THOUGHTS

The next time you find yourself procrastinating or feeling anxious or depressed about getting started on a task, activity, or chore, complete the following. It's best to do it as you're trying to start—while you're still in the situation—or as soon as possible thereafter so you don't forget important details.

1. **How are you feeling? (anxious, depressed, guilty, angry, etc.)**

   Anxious

2. **What is the current situation, event, task, or activity that you are faced with? What are you currently doing in the situation? (For example, responding to distractions—e.g., Internet, magazines, TV pacing around.) Be as descriptive as possible.**

   I am sitting down to continue work on an article that is due in 2 weeks. It is Wednesday

   afternoon. I am home alone. I feel I can't cope so I've been surfing the Web for sports news.

3. **Write down all the thoughts you are having in the situation—tune in particularly to thoughts you are having about *yourself.***

   I've been working on this article for 3 weeks and I've gotten nowhere on it. I should be able

   to dash off a piece like this quickly and easily. It is all over the place with no real point.

   It's terrible. I'll have to start all over again.

4. **Now, look back at your thoughts. What cognitive distortions do you recognize there? (Refer to your list and check off all those that apply.)**

   x   All-or-nothing thinking I have gotten nowhere on it . . . It's terrible.

   _____ Overgeneralization

   _____ Selective attention

   x   Disqualifying the positives I'll have to start all over again.

   _____ Personalization

   x   "Should" statements I should be able to dash off a piece like this quickly and easily.

   _____ Catastrophizing

(cont.)

Jumping to conclusions:

_____ Mind reading _____

_____ Fortune-teller error _____

5. Challenge these negative thoughts (distortions) by responding to the following questions that apply.

What is the evidence that the automatic thought is true?

Very little. The worst I can really say is that some of my submissions have needed

editing—but that's true of nearly all manuscripts on the first submission.

What is the evidence that the automatic thought is *not* true?

Actually, there's lots of evidence against these thoughts. I've only had one submission

rejected, and four articles published with positive feedback from the editor.

What's the worst that can happen?

The article could be rejected.

Could I live through it?

Yes, I'll have other opportunities.

What is the effect of my believing the automatic thought?

I'm procrastinating more.

What could be the effect of changing my thinking?

I could get started on a piece of it now and have a little less to do tomorrow.

6. What are more rational thoughts in response to the situation?

I've done good work before and I can do it again. Some parts of this article are good and

I will be able to use them. Right now I'm just going to do one section at a time and not

critique my work—I'll have time to review and edit it all at the end. Many good writers

write slowly.

7. Outcome—How do you feel now? How did the situation end?

A little more at ease—I could probably get started on an easy part.

LEADER NOTES

Time Management

Activation and Motivation

New Target Skills:
- Emotional distracters, continued (oppositionality).
- Self-activation.
- Distraction control.
- Visualization of rewards.

In-Session Exercise:
- Visualize rewards of achieving long-term goals.

Home Exercise:
- Visualize rewards of achieving long-term goals.

DEALING WITH EMOTIONAL DISTRACTERS (CONTINUED FROM PREVIOUS SESSION)

In addition to anxiety and depression (discussed last week) people with ADHD may find themselves **resistant or oppositional** to the demands, instructions, or expectations of others—particularly those in authority. This may occur as a result of a long history in which others (e.g., parents and teachers) were felt to constantly be imposing requirements and restrictions that were difficult, if not impossible, to meet.

Unfortunately, this attitude may persist in adulthood when the effect of resisting or opposing the methods of becoming more disciplined or more organized ultimately sabotages the person with ADHD and interferes with the attainment of his or her own cherished personal goals.

What to do when feeling oppositional? The feeling is usually experienced as **anger**.

Assess your thoughts and begin to challenge them.

What were you thinking when you became angry (feeling) and resistant (behavior)? Are the thoughts rational? What is the evidence that the thought is true?

Ask yourself whom are you doing it for. If it is not for you or for those you care about, you may need to reconsider your priorities. If the task is in line with your goals, resisting change will limit your control in the short run and prevent you from getting what you want in the long run. It will hurt you more than the "ghost" of authority.

For the rest of the session, we're going to focus on getting things done: (1) getting started or "activated," (2) overcoming distraction, and (3) staying on track toward long-term goals.

I. GET ACTIVATED

Do you remember the concept of the **"energy of activation"** from chemistry? That's the amount of energy, usually in the form of heat, that needs to be added to a chemical mixture before it will start to visibly react and give off heat, light, and so on. It's very similar in concept to the effort you have to put in to climb up to the top of a hill before you can take off and ski or sled down. Getting going on a task (particularly a boring, difficult one) is very much like that—you need to get oriented to it and get involved with it before you can "take off" and really make some headway with it.

Getting up that hill often seems to be particularly difficult for people with ADHD—the hill seems to be steeper and the effort more arduous. ***In fact, for people with ADHD, getting started is often the hardest part of the task!*** However, once at the top of the hill they may be able to ski down quite well! So, the focus needs to be on strategies to get the process going.

Some things that can be very useful are:

1. *Start small.* The real key is to do **something, anything**, however small. It may be as small as just gathering together the tools you will need for the repair job, or the files you will need to write the report.
2. *Start easy.* Begin with the **easiest** aspect of the task—one that you might even enjoy doing.
3. *Break it up into parts!*
4. *Plan a reward for yourself* to enjoy **after** the task is completed.
5. *Visualize yourself doing and completing the task:* If you want to remem-

ber to do something on your schedule, **visualize** yourself doing it at the appropriate time and place. For example: If you need to remember to take a pill as soon as you get home, imagine yourself opening your house door and going directly to the kitchen/bathroom to do it.

After taking the first step you can stop, pat yourself on the back, and decide **what** the next step will be and **when** you will take it. However, having gotten started, you may well have already built up some "energy of activation" and feel like continuing. If so, keep going! Before you do stop, however, be sure to decide when you will return to the task and what you will do next.

II. DISTRACTION CONTROL

Vulnerability to distraction is another big problem for people with ADHD. The distractions may be more immediate rewards and gratifications and they may also be **physical or social distractions.**

Avoiding Sensory Distractions

One of the keys to avoiding distractions is to "precommit" to working in a space that will be devoid of distractions. That may include the following:

1. Creating a workspace where there are **no visual distracters**—e.g., pictures, magazines, interesting books, and so on around you.

REMEMBER: *Out of sight, out of mind!*

----

2. Creating a workspace where there are **no auditory distracters.** Thus, be sure you:
   • Will not be able to hear the TV, other people talking, and so on when you are in your workspace.
   • If necessary, ask others to reduce those sounds while you are working.
   • Use headphones—with or without white noise.
   • Some types of music may be calming or focusing for some people with ADHD.
3. Another way to "precommit" is to **take yourself to another workspace** that you know in advance will be devoid of the distracters that tempt you most:
   • In college or graduate school, the library is often a good place to escape

social distractions, particularly in a room that is also far from interesting books and magazines.

- One young fellow I know who is a freelance writer and has ADHD knows that he must find a public space (e.g., library or coffee shop) that has *no free Internet access* if he hopes to accomplish anything on his writing while he is there.

Avoiding Social Distractions

Avoiding social distractions may be even harder than controlling physical distractions. It may be very tempting to chat with a friend or colleague when you know you should be working on that term paper or business report. Another difficulty in the office is that you may feel that your job demands that you be constantly available to others by phone, e-mail, or drop-in visit. Unless you are an EMS technician or work in an emergency room, this is very likely to be untrue! The reality is that if you fail to bracket some time for yourself, it will be extremely hard for you to get any other work done. You may set reasonable limits on your availability to others by instituting any or all of the following:

- Set up formal appointment hours when you are available for consultation or discussion.
- Hang a "Do Not Disturb" sign on your door.
- Ask your colleagues or family members to please not disturb you between certain hours and close your door.
- Turn off your phone ringer and let your answering machine take your calls.
- Close down your e-mail program and open it to check your e-mail only at predesignated times—for example, morning, midday, and end of day.

III. Sustaining Motivation

Short- versus Long-Term Reinforcers

Many of life's biggest rewards require long-term planning and effort. These rewards include saving for and purchasing a new home, earning an academic degree, winning a promotion, writing a book, composing a piece of music, and so on. When pursuing such long-term goals, it's easy to get bored, discouraged, or lose interest before the long-term rewards are achieved. ***This seems to be particularly true for people with ADHD for whom the long-term rewards don't seem to exert as much impact on how they go about their daily activities.*** Those rewards seem distant, remote, and unreal. Perhaps it is not surprising then, that those shadowy distant rewards easily get swamped when more immediate rewards present themselves.

So, for example, let's say you have a great idea that you'd like to work into a business proposal that would impress the boss and merit you a shot at a promotion. You make a plan to work on it on Saturday afternoon. Saturday, however, turns out to be a beautiful day and a friend calls you in the morning suggesting that you both go to the beach. This seems so much more appealing than sitting at a desk cooped up at home so you quickly accept and "poof" goes the idea of completing a project that could have helped you to advance at work, given you a new title, a raise, and more respect among your colleagues.

Increasing the Power of Distant Rewards

Suppose, however, someone had said to you at the moment of decision: "Now which would you really prefer—to go to the beach today or to become 'director' with a big raise and the corner office?" Undoubtedly, with that choice of small immediate versus major long-term rewards clearly before you, you would choose the latter (assuming, of course that you *want* to become the director!). The key, then, is to make those rewards feel more real and powerful in your mind in the **present**—so you can almost **taste** them—and therefore, choose the long-term reward over the immediate reward that will get you off course. We're going to discuss a strategy called **visualization of rewards** that will help you do just that.

You can help sustain the power of visualizing long-term rewards by keeping a visual image of your goal in nearby view—whether it be a picture of the corner office with a view, a mock-up of a book cover with your name as author, a new home, or a new wardrobe.

> NOTE TO THERAPIST: Some people with ADHD report the interesting phenomenon that they typically finish "90%" of a task, project, paper, or report, but do not complete it. There may be several possible reasons for this. Perfectionism may render the individual hesitant to call a job "finished" and/ or fearful of a negative evaluation of the final product. Another reason may be reluctance to start the next task, which is waiting immediately on the heels of the current one. Relatedly, the "devil"—that is, the problem/issue/task—you know is better than the one you don't! The therapist might ask participants to consider what they may be fearful of encountering after they finish and submit the final product.

In-Session Exercise: Visualization of Rewards

"Visualization of rewards" is a strategy to be used to assist yourself in getting started on and continuing work toward a cherished long-term goal, warding off distraction, diversion, and premature "giving up." **When you anticipate that you may have trouble getting started on the project, or when you feel tempted to quit, you take a few minutes to close your eyes and practice visualization of rewards.** In visualization of rewards, you mentally conjure up all the wonderful things and feelings you will have when you achieve your cherished goal.

At this point, solicit from the group a long-term goal one of them may have, have the group participants close their eyes, and together generate a list of the perks and positive feelings they will have access to when they achieve the long-term reward. The more concrete, visceral, and emotional the items, the better! If no one comes up with a goal, continue with the example above. Responses might include:

1. "Having my own parking space near the door."
2. "Getting a raise that would allow me to buy the home I've always wanted."
3. "Having my own full-time secretary."
4. "Being able to work on interesting projects of my own choosing."
5. "Having lunch in the executive dining room."
6. "Feeling great about myself."
7. "No longer having to take direction from [so-and-so]!"

Visualization of rewards works best **before** the temptation to choose the immediate reward arises. So, in the example above, if the individual wanted to be sure to work on the proposal on Saturday, he or she would do his or her **visualization of rewards** exercise first thing in the morning and then get to work on the proposal as soon as possible thereafter.

TAKE-HOME NOTES

Time Management
Activation and Motivation

Many people with ADHD know what they *should* do—for example, they may know *how* to be organized but they have trouble putting the strategies into effect—they have trouble getting started and maintaining motivation. This is often due to the unique difficulties that are characteristic of ADHD, especially vulnerability to distraction, boredom, and impatience, and low frustration tolerance. It may also be due to feelings of anger carried over from past relationships with authority figures. In this section we discuss strategies to address these difficulties.

I. DEALING WITH ANGER AND OPPOSITIONALITY

In addition to feelings of depression and anxiety, people with ADHD may find themselves **angry at "authority"** as a result of a long history in which others seemed to constantly impose requirements and restrictions that were difficult, if not impossible, to meet. Unfortunately, opposing authority in adulthood ultimately self-sabotages the person with ADHD and interferes with the attainment of his or her own cherished personal goals.

Begin to identify and challenge your thoughts when you find yourself getting angry or opposing changes that you've been wanting to make but just can't seem to.

For the rest of the session tonight, we are going to talk about how to get started on tasks, how to avoid distractions, and how to follow through to the end.

II. HOW TO GET STARTED AND STAY ON TRACK—TO THE FINISH LINE!

1. *Start small, start easy, break it down into parts.* It's essential when *planning* your schedule to break down any project into manageable "chunks" *and* plan a

(cont.)

---

reinforcement or reward for yourself after each "chunk." Examples are allowing yourself to watch a favorite TV show or read a chapter in that great mystery novel after you write each report. Checking off each item on your to-do list after you complete it is also very self-reinforcing.

2. ***Reinforcement must always be contingent.*** That is, you must **never** give yourself the reward unless you have completed the task.

3. ***Practice visualization.*** Take a few minutes to close your eyes and visualize yourself completing the task or project and how good/proud/satisfied/relieved you will feel then. It can be very powerfully motivating.

III. DEALING WITH DISTRACTIONS

Distractions can easily get you off track. But if you look out and plan for them, you can keep them from defeating you.

4. ***Know your work style and what works best for you***—then set the stage for success. If you do your best work uninterrupted, a few hours in the office at night or on the weekend may be better spent than a week working on a project when the phone calls keep coming in.

5. ***Use technology!*** Voice mail can answer your phone so you're not interrupted. Use headphones, possibly with white noise, if noise around your office or desk bothers you.

6. ***Keep distractions out of your field of vision—and hearing.*** Go somewhere to work where only the things needed for the job will be around you. For example, set up a study area at home where you don't have magazines, interesting books, and so on, and where you can't hear the TV or other people talking. Ask those in the house in advance not to interrupt you for *X* number of hours.

IV. SUSTAINING MOTIVATION OVER THE LONG TERM

People with ADHD are often tempted to choose the immediately gratifying reward over the longer-term or distant, but ultimately more satisfying, reward. For example, on a sunny Saturday in summer, you may choose to go to the beach rather than to stay in and follow through on your plan to work on a new business proposal, to complete a paper for a graduate course, or search for a better job. It is most important at these critical junctures to remind yourself—**and actively visualize**—all of the rewards in satisfaction, pride, and feelings of accomplishment, and the tangible rewards like money, or recognition, that you will experience once this larger project is completed.

TAKE-HOME EXERCISE

Time Management
Activation and Motivation

Step 1: Identify a long-term goal that you have wanted to achieve (e.g., finding a new job, renovating one or more rooms in your house, learning to play a musical instrument, writing a book or short story, pursuing a new project at work, etc.). By "long-term" we are referring to a goal that would reasonably take at least a month to achieve. Describe it here.

_____

_____

_____

Step 2: Think about a positive (but realistic) rewards scenario, including the feelings and experiences you will have when you achieve your goal. Write down the details here.

_____

_____

_____

_____

_____

_____

_____

_____

(cont.)

Step 3: Break down your long-term goal into a set of smaller, short-term (e.g., weekly) goals that you must achieve as steps along the way to your long-term goal. List them here.

1. _____

_____

2. _____

_____

3. _____

_____

4. _____

_____

5. _____

_____

Step 4: Schedule the first task, above, in your planner. Allow enough time to do the visualization.

Step 5: When the time comes to do the task, close your eyes and first visualize the long-term positive rewards as you have written them up in Step 2. Then complete the task.

Step 6: Write down the outcome. Did you complete the task? Did you visualize the rewards? Did visualization help motivate you to do the task?

_____

_____

_____

_____

_____

Step 7: Similarly schedule and complete the other items from Step 3. Write down the outcome(s).

_____

_____

_____

_____

_____

LEADER NOTES

Getting Organized

Setting Up an Organizational System

New Target Skill:

- Organizing a physical space for efficiency and reduction of distraction.

In-Session Exercise:

- Set up a filing system.
- Work through and diagram the organization of a physical space.

Take-Home Exercise:

- Organize one manageable part (A) of a larger personal physical space.

Materials:

- Manila folders with labels.

There are essentially two components to good organization:

1. *A place for everything and . . .*
2. *Everything in its place!*

The first component refers to the fact that there must be an organizational system or structure such that *everything "belongs" somewhere* and the second component refers to the fact that *everything must be put back in that place after use* if the system is to continue to operate. We discuss the first component today and the second component next time.

SETTING UP AN ORGANIZATIONAL SYSTEM

REMEMBER: *A place for everything!*

Why Be Organized?

Solicit ideas from group members. Be sure to highlight each of the following:

1. Can find things more easily.
2. Spend less *time* looking for things—can be more efficient.
3. Reduce stress.
4. Surroundings look more neat, attractive.

The Basics of an Organizational Plan

In a good organizational plan, everything must have a place that is

1. Easily identifiable.
2. Easily accessible.
3. Neat in appearance.

In addition, it is important for people with ADHD that the work space be *free of visual distracters* and that the items that are in immediate view are those that are related to the tasks at hand or otherwise *require* your attention.

Each room should be organized such that *the things you need to use most frequently are nearest at hand.* This may require a little thought, and it also may require the creation or purchase of containers, file drawers, baskets, or special boxes for storing and labeling particular groups of items. Think of the various functions or activities you undertake in each space. For example, in your study, let's say you

1. Take care of personal finances.
2. Read or write materials related to your job.
3. Pursue a hobby, such as photography or sewing.

Julie Morgenstern, who has written a helpful book on personal organization (Morgenstern, 2004), suggests you create a "zone" in the room for each of these functions, with all the relevant materials. For example, in an area that is devoted to management of finances, you would include the files for your bank accounts, credit card statements, utility bills, home rental or mortgage expenses, and a drawer in which to keep your checkbook, calculator, and so on. The zone for your job-related activities would probably include your computer, printer, and the files related to your work. The zone for your hobby would have all the supplies and equipment you need for that activity grouped together. You might even make a diagram to plan out how you will organize the space.

Creating a Filing System

All papers should be in **manila file folders that are clearly labeled** and filed upright in file drawers or in vertical files on your desktop **in alphabetical order** for easy relocation. It's very helpful to use **color coding** for quick finding (e.g., all financial folders are green in color, all hobbies/personal interest folders are in blue).

In-Session Exercise 1: Setting Up a Filing System

Ask participants to come up with names for file labels for the kinds of papers they need to file. Prompt them when necessary using the following. Show them several file folders already labeled and demonstrate how they would be filed in alphabetical order.

Examples of file folder labels:

Personal interest	Personal business
Health	Bank of New York (for statements)
Gardening	Visa (for statements)
Home Decorating	Mortgage
Gift Ideas	Legal Documents (birth and marriage certificates, will, etc.)
Housewares (instruction booklets, warranties)	Auto Insurance
Articles of Interest	Home Insurance

Family History	Taxes 2011 (statements, receipts, etc., needed for filing)
Photography	Medical Insurance
Travel	Retirement
Home Improvement	Receipts from Recently Purchased Items

In-Box and Out-Box

It's also very helpful to keep on your desk an **"in-box"** (or in-folder) for incoming bills and letters that require a response, and an **"out-box"** for completed letters that have to be mailed or other material that has to be moved to a different room, taken to work and so on. In-box items should be taken care of at least once per week at a designated time (e.g., every Saturday morning). Out-box items should be moved on to their final destination when you leave your desk after that session.

The Process

Organizing a physical space, particularly one that is piled high with clutter, is a very demanding job that can feel quite aversive. The strategies we have discussed to get started and follow through on difficult tasks are useful here as well:

1. *Divide the task into parts.* Don't expect to be able to organize your entire study or garage at one time. Instead, divide it up into parts (e.g., divide the space into a grid, and work on one section at a time), or plan to spend just 30 minutes at a time (or however much you feel you can tolerate). Set a timer if it makes you feel better, knowing there will be a definite end to the process.

2. Based on the above, *decide how many "sessions" you will need altogether and make a list*—assigning a date and time to each. Schedule the sessions in your planner.

3. Plan to give yourself a (well-earned) **reinforcer** after each part.

4. As soon as you feel tempted to stop, close your eyes and **visualize** how well the space will look and function when it is neat and organized and how good you will feel about it (and yourself).

5. *Use a system to sort* out what is worth keeping and what should be thrown out. An easy-to-remember concept is **"FAT"—File–Action–Trash**. Set up three

cardboard boxes (or three large plastic bags) with one of these labels. Every item that passes through your hands should go into one of these three boxes, depending upon whether it needs to be **filed**/saved/put away, whether some **action** has to be taken with it, or whether it should be thrown into the **trash**. Don't spend much time debating. If you can't quickly decide what to do with it, put it in the action box to reconsider later.

6. If possible, *enlist the help of someone* who will be supportive as you go through the process.

Caution! When going through interesting materials you may be very tempted to stop and read that newspaper clipping, or reread that letter from a friend, or look through that catalog . . . **Resist the urge** . . . *otherwise you may well get sidetracked and never finish your task*. Instead, set aside those interesting materials to look at when you take a break—for example, make it your reinforcer (Step 3 above).

In-Session Exercise 2

Solicit from the group a physical space (e.g., study, garage, den, kitchen, closet) that needs to be organized. With group input, make a diagram on the board of how the space could be organized, considering the items currently in the space, the functions that need to occur there, matters of convenience, ease of access, and so on. Consider also the organizational tools (e.g., file folders, upright file holders, bins, drawer organizers) that might be useful.

> NOTE TO THERAPIST: Some individuals with ADHD say that they are reluctant to become organized because they perceive organized people to be "boring" or "rigid," and they are afraid of losing their spontaneity and creativity. While there is surely more than a modicum of post hoc rationalization of the status quo here, it may also be the case that being organized and planful feels so alien to the ADHD sufferer that there is a fear of loss of some essential characteristic of his or her personality. In addressing this concern, it is important to emphasize and illustrate that, far from creating additional constraints, better organization of the mundane aspects of daily living will allow the individual many more opportunities to freely develop, express, and enjoy his or her essential and unique gifts, talents, and interests.

TAKE-HOME NOTES

Getting Organized
Setting Up an Organizational System

REMEMBER: *A place for everything!*

The Plan

In a good organizational plan, everything must have a place that is

1. Easily identifiable.
2. Easily accessible.
3. Neat in appearance.

In addition, it is important for people with ADHD that the work space be **free of visual distracters** and that the items that are in immediate view are those that are related to the tasks at hand or otherwise *require* your attention.

 Each room should be organized such that *the things you need to use most frequently are nearest at hand*. This may require a little thought, and it also may require the creation or purchase of containers, file drawers, baskets, or special boxes for storing and labeling particular groups of items. Think of the various functions or activities you undertake in each space. For example, in your study, let's say you

1. Take care of personal finances.
2. Read or write materials related to your job.
3. Pursue a hobby, such as photography or sewing.

(cont.)

Julie Morgenstern, who has written a helpful book on personal organization (Morgenstern, 2004), suggests you create a "zone" in the room for each of these functions, with all the relevant materials. For example, in an area that is devoted to management of finances, you would include the files for your bank accounts, credit card statements, utility bills, home rental or mortgage expenses, and a drawer in which to keep your checkbook, calculator, and so on. The zone for your job-related activities would probably include your computer, printer, and the files related to your work. The zone for your hobby would have all the supplies and equipment you need for that activity grouped together. You might even make a diagram to plan out how you will organize the space.

Creating a Filing System

All papers should be in **manila file folders that are clearly labeled** and filed upright in file drawers or in vertical files on your desktop **in alphabetical order** for easy location. It's very helpful to use **color coding** for quick finding (e.g., all financial folders are green in color, all hobbies/personal interest folders are in blue).

In-Box and Out-Box

It's also very helpful to keep on your desk an **"in-box"** (or in-folder) for incoming bills and letters that require a response, and an **"out-box"** for completed letters that have to be mailed or other material that has to be moved to a different room, taken to work, and so on. In-box items should be taken care of at least once per week at a designated time (e.g., every Saturday morning). Out-box items should be moved on to their final destination when you leave your desk after that session.

The Process

Organizing a physical space, particularly one that is piled high with clutter, is a very demanding job that can feel quite aversive. The strategies we have discussed to get started and follow through on difficult tasks are useful here as well:

1. **Divide the task into parts.** Don't expect to be able to organize your entire study or garage at one time. Instead, divide it up into parts (e.g., divide the space into a grid, and work on one section at a time), or plan to spend just 30 minutes at a time (or however much you feel you can tolerate). Set a timer if it makes you feel better, knowing there will be a definite end to the process.

2. Based on the above, **decide how many "sessions" you will need altogether and make a list**—assigning a date and time to each. Schedule the sessions in your planner.

3. Plan to give yourself a (well-earned) **reinforcer** after each part.

(cont.)

162

4. As soon as you feel tempted to stop, close your eyes and **visualize** how well the space will look and function when it is neat and organized and how good you will feel about it (and yourself).

5. *Use a system to sort* out what is worth keeping and what should be thrown out. An easy-to-remember concept is **"FAT"—File–Action–Trash**. Set up three cardboard boxes (or three large plastic bags) with one of these labels. Every item that passes through your hands should go into one of these three boxes, depending upon whether it needs to be **filed**/saved/put away, whether some **action** has to be taken with it, or whether it should be thrown into the **trash**. Don't spend much time debating. If you can't quickly decide what to do with it, put it in the action box to reconsider later.

6. If possible, *enlist the help of someone* who will be supportive as you go through the process.

Caution! When going through interesting materials you may be very tempted to stop and read that newspaper clipping, or reread that letter from a friend, or look through that catalog . . . *Resist the urge . . . otherwise you may well get sidetracked and never finish your task*. Instead, set aside those interesting materials to look at when you take a break—for example, make it your reinforcer (Step 3 above).

TAKE-HOME EXERCISE

Getting Organized
Setting Up an Organizational System

Step 1: Choose one physical space where you would like to be more organized or function more efficiently—for example, home study, office, kitchen, closet, tool shed, car (the possibilities are endless!).

Step 2: Divide the space into three manageable parts and make a list of these below.

Step 3: Choose one part and then, employing the principles previously discussed in this session, **plan** how you will reorganize that space. Be sure to take time to **think** about your approach and write up your **plan** below or make a diagram before you jump in. You will do another part next time.

REMEMBER: *If you're having trouble getting started, you've started out on too big a level.* Scale it down further (e.g., reorganize one shelf first instead of the whole closet, or organize the glove compartment instead of the whole car).

Step 4 (optional but recommended): **Take "before" and "after" photos so you can see the results of your work!**

Space: _____

Parts:

A. _____

B. _____

C. _____

(cont.)

Plan of action for Part A: _____

_____

_____

_____

_____

_____

_____

What I accomplished: _____

_____

_____

_____

_____

_____

_____

LEADER NOTES

Getting Organized

Implementing an Organizational System

New Target Skill:

- Following through on organization of a physical space, applying self-management techniques.

In-Session Exercises:

- Sort paper pile.
- Designate locations for frequently misplaced items

Take-Home Exercise:

- Organize Part B of physical space.

Materials:

- Bag of miscellaneous mail, papers, etc.

NOTE TO THERAPIST: No new material will be introduced in this session (and there are no Take-Home Notes) in order to allow sufficient time to discuss each participant's Take-Home Exercise, eliciting his or her main organizational needs and objectives and assisting in the selection and development of the appropriate system, applying the principles discussed in the previous session.

If participants appear to be having difficulty with follow-through on their organizational plans, review "The Process" section from Session 7 and reinvoke specific skills from earlier sessions such as breaking down difficult tasks into manageable chunks, contingent self-reinforcement, and visualization of rewards (in this case, visualizing the order, ease, and efficiency that will result from having a neat, organized space).

IN-SESSION EXERCISE 1: SORT PAPER PILE

Bring in a bag of miscellaneous papers, mail, and so on of the type that typically accumulates and needs to be sorted and filed or thrown out—perhaps obtained from your or a colleagues' desk (excluding confidential documents, of course). This exercise can be led either by the therapist or (preferably) by one or more volunteers from the group taking turns. The exercise is to sort the mail, item by item in front of the group, holding up and describing each piece, and asking the group's input as to what should be done with each (file, action, or trash; if filed, under what file name).

IN-SESSION EXERCISE 2

Solicit from the group a list of items that are repeatedly lost or misplaced (e.g., keys, cell phone, receipts, documents needed for taxes) and develop easy-to-find locations for them. For example, a hook for keys may be mounted near the door.

TAKE-HOME EXERCISE

The Take-Home Exercise is to continue working on the next part or "zone" of the organizational plan.

TAKE-HOME EXERCISE

Getting Organized
Implementing an Organizational System

Step 1: Go back to last week's exercise and choose Part B to reorganize this time.

Step 2: Employing the principles in Session 7, **plan** how you will reorganize this space. Be sure to take time to **think** about your approach and write up your **plan** below or make a diagram before you jump in.

Step 3: Reorganize the space using the principles we discussed.

Plan of action for Part B:

_____

_____

_____

_____

_____

What I accomplished:

_____

_____

_____

_____

_____

Getting Organized

Maintaining an Organizational System

New Target Skill:
- Maintaining organization.

In-Session Exercise:
- Work through a plan to maintain organization.

Take-Home Exercise:
- Sort the mail.
- Organize Part C of physical space.

REMEMBER: . . . *Everything in its place!*

This is probably the hardest part of organization for people with ADHD. Putting things in their place after use and filing away new items as they come in, is probably one of the least rewarding tasks of daily life! It's boring, tedious, and not immediately gratifying—all attributes that make it *most* unappealing to people with ADHD. But it is essential to maintaining **order,** which is necessary for just about everything **else** you may want to do.

The most important key for dealing with this is to *not let things pile up*. The "things" may be mail, dishes, papers to be sorted and filed, clothes, and other personal belongings. Seeing a pile of things that need to be dealt with is most discouraging, overwhelming, and, you *know*, will require *long* effort before any results are seen. Most likely, therefore, you will never want to even start, and the pile will grow even larger day by day . . . and you will be even *less* likely to want to touch it, and the pile will grow even *larger* day by day . . . (repeat, repeat ad nauseam).

The most successful approach, therefore, is to ***put things away on an immediate or daily basis*. Why do it?** The advantages are:

1. You will *always* easily be able to find the things you need.
2. The place will *always* appear neat and tidy. Although you may not be fully aware of it, the appearance of disorder and disorganization is *stressful*.
3. Each tidying/putting away effort will only last *a few minutes* and then you will have the (nearly immediate) gratification of seeing a positive result— the desk will be *clear*, the kitchen will be *clean*.

REMEMBER: *What you don't do today won't go away—*
it will just be that much harder tomorrow!

DEALING WITH THE MAIL

Mail is a perfect example of something that takes only a few minutes to deal with on a daily basis, but, when neglected, can accumulate to overwhelming proportions. Here is a strategy to deal with it.

What is the first thing you do when you get home? Get something to eat? Sink down on the couch and flip on the TV? The suggestion here is to put off those things for **just *a few minutes*** while you deal with the mail, and **then** you can relax.

1. Shortly after you get in the house, go through the mail while you **stand or sit next to a wastebasket**.
2. Immediately throw away **unwanted items** (e.g., ads, circulars).
3. Sort the remaining items into bills to be paid, statements and other information to be filed, and so on, and **immediately place the items in their appropriate folders**. Items that need further action (e.g., letters needing a response) should be put into your in-box.
4. Enter any new items for social engagements, appointments, and so on in

your planner or on the calendar. Be sure to include the time, location, and directions for getting there, as well as other requirements (e.g., dress). Also enter into your planner anything you need to do in advance for the event—for example, enter the date on which you will buy the gift, shop for the outfit to wear, call the babysitter, and so on.

And you're done! If you don't believe it's that quick, I'd like you to time yourself tonight or tomorrow when you next get your mail. (Note that this is the first part of the Take-Home Exercise.)

Note: If it proves too difficult to file things away immediately, then at least get them into your in-box and sit down religiously (e.g., every Saturday or Sunday morning at a specified time) and deal with every item in your in-box.

Hot tax tip: You'll save yourself much time and aggravation come April if you keep a folder by your desk to file all your relevant receipts for tax-deductible items—*Just stick them in the folder as they come into the house!*

Bill-paying tip: Online banking is an enormous time-saver. It takes only about an hour to set it up initially and you'll never have to spend time making out checks, recording, and mailing them again. You can even set it up to generate fixed monthly checks on an automatic basis (e.g., car payment, mortgage) so you won't have to worry about forgetting.

IN-SESSION EXERCISE: MAINTAINING ORGANIZATION

Solicit from the group another problem that needs to be tackled (doing the dishes, putting away clothes, tools, etc.) and work through a system for dealing with it on a **daily** basis.

NOTE TO THERAPIST: Even if it is not offered by a group member, mention here the need to take the last few minutes of the day at work to put away materials, file papers, and so on so that the next morning one comes in to a clear desk ready to begin work anew. Accumulated piles of material on the desk is a great problem for many people with ADHD.

TAKE-HOME NOTES

Getting Organized

Maintaining an Organizational System

REMEMBER: *. . . Everything in its place!*

The most important key for dealing with this is to *not let things pile up.* The "things" may be mail, dishes, papers to be sorted and filed, clothes, and other personal belongings. Seeing a pile of things that need to be dealt with is most discouraging, overwhelming, and, you *know*, will require *long* effort before any results are seen. Most likely, therefore, you will never want to even start, and the pile will grow even larger day by day . . . and you will be even *less* likely to want to touch it, and the pile will grow even *larger* day by day . . . (repeat, repeat ad nauseam).

REMEMBER: *What you don't do today won't go away—*
it will just be that much harder tomorrow!

DEALING WITH THE MAIL

Mail is a perfect example of something that takes only a few minutes to deal with on a daily basis, but, when neglected, can accumulate to overwhelming proportions. Here is a strategy to deal with it.

What is the first thing you do when you get home? Get something to eat? Sit down on the couch and flip on the TV? The suggestion here is to put off those things for **just a few minutes** while you deal with the mail, and **then** you can relax.

(cont.)

1. Shortly after you get in the house, go through the mail while you **stand or sit next to a wastebasket**.
2. Immediately throw away **unwanted items** (e.g., ads, circulars).
3. Sort the remaining items into bills to be paid, statements and other information to be filed, and so on, and *immediately place the items in their appropriate folders*. Items that need further action (e.g., letters needing a response) should be put into your in-box.
4. Enter any new items for **social engagements**, appointments, and so on in your planner or on the calendar. Be sure to include the time, location, and directions for getting there, as well as other requirements (e.g., dress). Also enter into your planner anything you need to do in advance for the event—for example, enter the date on which you will buy the gift, shop for the outfit to wear, call the babysitter, and so on.

And you're done! If you don't believe it's that quick, I'd like you to *time* yourself tonight or tomorrow when you next get your mail. (Note that this is the first part of the Take-Home Exercise.)

Note: If it proves too difficult to file things away immediately, then at least get them into your in-box and sit down religiously (e.g., every Saturday or Sunday morning at a specified time) and deal with every item in your in-box.

Hot tax tip: You'll save yourself much time and aggravation come April if you keep a folder by your desk to file all your relevant receipts for tax-deductible items—*Just stick them in the folder as they come into the house!*

Bill-paying tip: Online banking is an enormous time-saver. It takes only about an hour to set it up initially and you'll never have to spend time making out checks, recording, and mailing them again. You can even set it up to generate fixed monthly checks on an automatic basis (e.g., car payment, mortgage) so you won't have to worry about forgetting.

TAKE-HOME EXERCISE

Getting Organized
Maintaining an Organizational System

TAKE-HOME EXERCISE 1: SORTING THE MAIL

Time yourself dealing with your mail using the system we discussed today.

Write down: Start time: _____ Finish time: _____

Try to use the system every day this week. Check below each day that you use it.

Monday	Tuesday	Wednesday	Thursday	Friday	Saturday

TAKE-HOME EXERCISE 2: ORGANIZE PART C

Step 1: Go back to Session 7's exercise and choose Part C to reorganize this time.

Step 2: Employing the principles in Session 7, **plan** how you will reorganize this space. Be sure to take time to **think** about your approach and write up your **plan** below or make a diagram before you jump in.

Step 3: Reorganize the space using the principles we discussed.

Step 4: Come up with a plan for **maintaining** the organization you create for this zone.

Step 5: Take your "after" photo and, if you'd like, bring it to group to share!

(cont.)

Plan of action for Part C:

_____

_____

_____

_____

_____

_____

_____

What I accomplished:

_____

_____

_____

_____

_____

_____

Plan for maintaining organization of this space:

_____

_____

_____

_____

_____

_____

_____

_____

Plan a Project—and Get It Done!

New Target Skill:
- Planning a project utilizing the skills of breakdown of tasks into sub-tasks, prioritizing, scheduling, visualization of rewards, sustaining motivation, self-reward, and enlisting others' support.

In-Session Exercise:
- Plan a project with a "flowchart."

Take-Home Exercise:
- Plan a project with a "flowchart" (with sample).

Planning a project and completing it incorporates many of the skills we have discussed concerning time estimation and scheduling, prioritizing, breaking down a larger task into manageable chunks, and sustaining motivation by self-reward, visualization of rewards, and so on. It all comes together here! In order to illustrate the process, let's select a project that one of you is currently planning or would like to accomplish.

IN-SESSION EXERCISE

Solicit examples from the group. Home-based projects such as small renovations or decorating, party planning, or planning a vacation work best. If a work project is chosen, solicit enough details to make sure it is not too technical for the group to work on.

If no project is suggested by the group, then use the following: "Plan a dinner party for 12 people." (Alternatively, "Plan a vacation trip.") A more challenging example would be to plan a dinner meeting of 100 people, with a speaker, for your alumni group/club/social organization.

Hand out copies of the project planning "flowchart" (the second part of the Take-Home Exercise) and make a copy on the whiteboard as you work. Explain the process of breaking down the main goal into successive sets of subgoals. Work out the first set of subgoals with input from group participants. For example, planning a dinner party would require selecting the date and then deciding on the guest list, menu, table decor, and home preparation (one per box). In the third column, break down each of these still further (e.g., planning the guest list requires purchasing, addressing, and mailing the invitations). Travel planning requires deciding on the date and destination, and then (one per box) making reservations for train or airline, reserving the hotel, deciding what to pack, making home arrangements for pet sitting, mail collection, and so on. Planning the dinner meeting would require knowing the budget available, and then planning for each of the following (one to a box): choice of speaker, choice of site, invitations, and on-site preparations. Each of these would then have subgoals, which the therapist would similarly work out with input from group participants and then indicate all on the whiteboard in the appropriate boxes. The date of the dinner meeting may be fixed or may depend on mutual availability of the speaker, site, and so on. Be sure to assign a completion date to each subgoal. A fourth column may be added to the flowchart for more ambitious or complex projects.

At each step, be sure to question the participants regarding what is involved in completing the task/subgoal—especially what information, materials, and assistance of others will be needed and how these may be obtained. Each of these would then constitute subgoals.

After completing the flowchart, solicit comments from participants about where they might expect difficulties in the process to occur (or have typically occurred for them in the past) and troubleshoot these problems with group input.

TAKE-HOME EXERCISE

Help each participant choose a personal project to work on during the coming 2 weeks using the flowchart. Be sure that the projects are modest ones that can easily be completed in 2 weeks—or even in 1 week. As time permits, help participants get started on their flowcharts for their respective projects.

TAKE-HOME EXERCISE

Plan a Project—and Get It Done!

Select a project that you will plan and begin in the next week, and complete the following week.

Step 1: Complete the flowchart on the next page for the project, using the same procedures that we used in the session. Be sure to insert dates for completion of each task.

Step 2: Review the items you have written in the right-hand column. In each box, assign a priority number to each item. Start again with number "1" in each new box. Also write in the tasks you will ask for help with and the name of the person you will ask to help you.

Step 3: Schedule a time slot in your planner in which you will take care of each of the items that need to be done for the project during the coming week. *Schedule the highest priority items from each box first and then schedule the other items.* Note that an "item" can be as simple as a phone call to get information or to ask someone to help you with a task. When possible, try to include the tasks in your daily routine so you don't have to make too many "special trips." For example, if you need to buy invitations and you know they are sold at your supermarket, put them on your shopping list of items to get when you next go to the supermarket.

Step 4: As you complete each item, check it off on your flowchart and in your planner. (It's a good feeling!)

Step 5: Make a note here of any problems you encountered in planning for or carrying out the project. There will be an opportunity to share and discuss these at the next group meeting.

_____

_____

_____

_____

(cont.)

PROJECT PLANNING
FLOWCHART

Date Due: _____

Budget:

Target Date: _____

Target Date: _____

Target Date: _____

Target Date: _____

SAMPLE OF A COMPLETED FLOWCHART

Dinner party for 12 people

Date Due: 6/15

Budget:

Guest list

Target Date: 4/15

Update address book 4/1
Purchase invitations and stamps 4/5
Address invitations 4/7
Mail invitations 4/15

Menu

Target Date: 5/15

Review magazines and cookbooks 4/16
Finalize menu 4/20
Purchase dry goods 6/1
Purchase fresh goods 6/12 and 6/13
Prepare menu 6/13, 6/14, and 6/15

Decor

Target Date: 5/30

Research party tents 5/13
Research gardeners 5/13
Schedule gardener 5/15
Purchase centerpiece, tablecloths, etc. 5/13
Schedule tent delivery 5/30

Home preparation

Target Date: 6/14

Clean cutlery and china 6/7 and 6/8
Clean house 6/10 and 6/11

180

LEADER NOTES

Project Planning

Implementation

New Target Skills:
- Applying self-management techniques previously discussed to ensure continued implementation of plan for project.

In-Session Exercise:
- Review progress on participants' projects.

Take-Home Exercise:
- Complete personal project.

NOTE TO THERAPIST: No new material is planned for today in order to allow adequate time to discuss each participant's project. There are no Take-Home Notes nor new Take-Home Exercise.

In discussing each participant's project, take care to incorporate and emphasize the skills listed in previous sections wherever possible—for example, allocating regular time to the project in one's planner, prioritizing within the day, adhering to deadlines for subgoals, using techniques such as visualization of rewards, and enlisting support of others to sustain motivation through to completion.

TAKE-HOME EXERCISE

Continue work on the project, completing it in the coming week.

Looking to the Future

Goals:
- Help the participants to:
  - Self-evaluate their progress in the program, their current status, and future needs.
  - Formulate a specific plan to meet future needs.
  - Express feelings about termination.
  - Complete formal postgroup self-evaluations and program evaluation.

Take-Home Notes:
- Looking to the future.

I. SELF-EVALUATION

Highlight that participants came to the group at different stages on their growth journey, that each responded to the program differently, and that each now is at a different "place" with respect to needs and goals. Go around the room, after the review of the Take-Home Exercise, and invite participants to share with the group where they are now in terms of their personal journey—goals achieved, and goals desired.

> **NOTE TO THERAPIST:** This is an important opportunity for the therapist to highlight and reinforce positive changes, including new strategies learned, habits changed, and insights attained. In the roundtable discussion, the therapist can actively highlight these in instances in which the participant omits or devalues them.

II. SUGGEST OPTIONS FOR CONTINUED GROWTH

These may include individual therapy, coaching, and future groups. Anticipate with the participants what difficulties might arise in the future and how these might be recognized and addressed.

At an appropriate point during the session, review aloud with participants the summary of strategies in "Looking to the Future" in the Take-Home Notes.

III. ELICIT FEELINGS ABOUT TERMINATION

Ask group participants how they have felt about the group, and how they are feeling now that it is ending. This discussion may lead to interest in a future group or "booster" sessions.

IV. COMPLETION OF PERSONAL EVALUATION MATERIALS AND PROGRAM EVALUATION

To evaluate the progress of group participants, allow the last 30–45 minutes of the session to have participants complete the CAARS, BRIEF, ON-TOP, Beck Depression Inventory, and any other questionnaires completed at baseline. Have each also complete a participant evaluation of the program.

TAKE-HOME NOTES

Looking to the Future

The following is a summary of the key strategies we have discussed—suitable for posting.

BREAK IT DOWN

Break each task down into parts.

If you're still having trouble getting started, break it down into even smaller parts.

Schedule each task in your planner; estimate how long it will take; prioritize.

If it's not in your planner, it doesn't exist.

Plan a pleasurable little reward for completing each task.

For ideas, consult your personal renewal list from Session 3.

Visualize completing the task.

Imagine all the pleasurable feelings and results that will follow.

Time yourself as you complete each task.

Compare your actual time to your estimated time to hone your judgment of how long things take.

(cont.)

GETTING STARTED IS THE HARDEST PART

Ease your way into the task by starting with the easiest part.

If you're still having trouble getting started, you're planning to do too much.

Never leave off a task at a difficult point; it will be harder to start again.

If you can't decide what to do first, do the next priority item in your planner.

To narrow it down further:

- Do the thing that you are *least* likely to do.
- Do the thing that's most *convenient* at the moment.
- Do the thing that you would most *enjoy* doing right now.

Minimize distractions.

Go where you don't have interesting magazines or books around. Don't have TV, radio, or people talking within earshot. Close your door. Use voice mail to intercept calls.

GET ORGANIZED

Choose a space to organize and break it down into "zones."

If you're still having trouble getting started, break down the zone into even smaller parts.

Have a plan of action for each zone.

Use the FAT system for decision making—File, Action, or Trash. When filing or storing things, subtract before you add. Partner with a friend. Use music.

Maintain the zone. Don't let the task get daunting again!

It's easier to keep a rolling stone in motion than it is to move it for the first time.

Getting to Bed, Getting Up, and Getting to Work on Time

New Target Skills:
- Understanding the reasons why participants might have difficulty getting up and to work on time.
- Developing strategies to address these problems.

Take-Home Exercise:
- Identify your thoughts.
- Track your progress.

Being late to work is a common problem for adults with ADHD. However, you can't get to work on time if you don't get up on time, and you can't get up on time if you don't get to bed on time. So that's where we begin!

I. WHY IS GETTING TO BED HARD FOR MANY PEOPLE WITH ADHD?

First solicit answers from the participants and write them on the whiteboard. Be sure to add the following to the list if not spontaneously given by the group:

186

- It's hard to stop what you're doing (e.g., stimulating behaviors like surfing the Web, playing video games, reading, TV).
- You finally have "alone time" to enjoy or to finish work (because time is not well planned during the day, etc.).
- Erratic bedtime and wake time means that you don't feel sleepy when it's time to go to bed.

II. WHAT ARE THE PROBLEMS CAUSED BY NOT GETTING TO BED ON TIME?

Detail the physical and mental consequences of insufficient sleep. Include fatigue, vulnerability to physical illness, and negative effects on many of the same functions (focused and sustained attention, organization, etc.) that are already compromised in people with ADHD.

III. WHAT CAN YOU DO TO PROMOTE A CONSISTENT BEDTIME?

1. **Have a distinct bedtime and stick to it** (with *a little* variation allowed on weekends). The body gets used to a distinct bedtime and cooperates by getting sleepy at about that time. Most adults need 7–9 hours of sleep per night.

2. Plan to start relaxing and get ready for bed an hour before bedtime.
   - **That means turning OFF sources of stimulation, including:**
     - Turn off the computer.
     - Turn off the cell phone.
     - Turn off the TV.
     - Try to avoid exercise or a heavy meal within a couple of hours before bedtime.
   - **It means turning ON sources of relaxation, including:**
     - Take a warm bath.
     - Turn on relaxing music.
     - Take a book to bed (but not one that you won't be able to put down!).

3. People often resist going to bed because it's the first time during the day that they can do exactly what they want to do—with no demands by employers, spouses, children, or others. One solution to this is to allow more "downtime" or "me-time" during the day/early evening (i.e., stop the work sooner).

4. If you're still having trouble **stopping** so as to get ready for bed, make a list on an index card of the consequences of staying up too late—how you'll feel, look,

and perform tomorrow, and keep it on the pillow, bedside table, or other prominent place where you can view it when you are most likely to be "hyperfocused."

5. Solicit other solutions from the group.

IV. What Can You Do to Promote Consistent Wake-Up and Getting to Work on Time?

1. By getting to bed on time, you have already gone a long way toward ensuring that you will be able to get up on time—refreshed and with energy to **go**!

2. **Plan** your morning predeparture routine.
- Know exactly how much time you need (if necessary, do a time estimation) to get ready **comfortably but efficiently,** without a frantic rush, and how much travel time you must allow.
- Plan whatever you can the night before:
  - *Consult your planner* to see what you have to do the next day.
  - Select clothes.
  - Make lunch.
  - Gather items in your briefcase or bag that must be brought with you, and place by the door.

3. **Set an alarm**—or two, if necessary. If you've gotten enough sleep, you may not even need the alarm.

In-Session Exercise: My Arguments for Going to Bed on Time

Pass out 4 × 6″ index cards and ask the participants to write down their personal reasons for getting to bed on time: e.g., "I will be better able to concentrate tomorrow," "I will be more efficient at work," "I won't feel exhausted and irritable." The participants should make the strongest case possible for the benefits of getting to bed on time. The cards will be used during the home exercise, as described below.

TAKE-HOME NOTES

Getting to Bed, Getting Up, and Getting to Work on Time

Being late to work is a common problem for adults with ADHD. However, you can't get to work on time if you don't get up on time, and you can't get up on time if you don't get to bed on time. So that's where we begin!

I. WHY IS GETTING TO BED HARD FOR MANY PEOPLE WITH ADHD?

- It's hard to stop what you're doing (e.g., stimulating behaviors like surfing the Web, playing video games, reading, TV).
- You finally have alone time to enjoy (because time is not well planned during the day, etc.).
- Erratic bedtime and wake time means that you don't feel sleepy when it's time to go to bed.

II. WHAT ARE THE PROBLEMS CAUSED BY NOT GETTING TO BED ON TIME?

These include fatigue, vulnerability to physical illness, and negative effects on many of the same functions (focused and sustained attention, organization, etc.) that are already compromised in people with ADHD.

III. WHAT CAN YOU DO TO PROMOTE A CONSISTENT BEDTIME?

1. **Have a distinct bedtime and stick to it** (with a *little* variation allowed on weekends). The body gets used to a distinct time and cooperates by getting sleepy at about that time. Most adults need 7–9 hours of sleep per night.

(cont.)

Note: If you've gotten used to going to bed very late, and would like to be able to get up earlier, set your clock earlier by a small amount (e.g., 15 minutes) each morning. And similarly, plan to go to bed that much earlier each night. If you continue to get up earlier, you will become tired earlier in the evening and better able to go to sleep.

2. Plan to start relaxing and get ready for bed an hour before bedtime.
- **That means turning OFF sources of stimulation, including:**
  - Turn off the computer.
  - Turn off the cell phone.
  - Turn off the TV.
  - Try to avoid exercise or a heavy meal within a couple of hours before bedtime.
- **It means turning ON sources of relaxation, including:**
  - Take a warm bath.
  - Turn on relaxing music.
  - Take a book to bed (but not one that you won't be able to put down!).

3. People often people resist going to bed because it's the first time during the day that they can do exactly what they want to do—with no demands by employers, spouses, children, or others. One solution to this is to allow more "downtime" or "me-time" during the day/early evening (i.e., stop the work sooner).

4. If you're still having trouble **stopping** so as to get ready for bed, make a list on an index card of the consequences of staying up too late—how you'll feel, look, and perform tomorrow, and keep it on the pillow, bedside table, or other prominent place where you can view it when you are most likely to be "hyperfocused."

IV. WHAT CAN YOU DO TO PROMOTE CONSISTENT WAKE-UP AND GETTING TO WORK ON TIME?

1. By getting to bed on time, you have already gone a long way toward ensuring that you will be able to get up on time—refreshed and with energy to **go**!

2. **Plan** your morning predeparture routine.
- Know exactly how much time you need (if necessary, do a time estimation) to get ready **comfortably but efficiently**, without a frantic rush, and how much travel time you must allow.
- Plan whatever you can the night before:
  - *Consult your planner* to see what you have to do the next day.
  - Select clothes.
  - Make lunch.
  - Gather items in your briefcase or bag that must be brought with you, and place by the door.

3. **Set an alarm**—or two, if necessary. If you've gotten enough sleep, you may not even need the alarm.

TAKE-HOME EXERCISE

Getting to Bed, Getting Up, and Getting to Work on Time

Step 1: Plan. Considering the issues we have discussed in this session, decide what time it would be best for you to get to **sleep**. Allow **an hour** before that time to begin bedtime preparations, and to get into "relaxation mode."

If you've gotten used to going to bed very late, and would like to be able to get up earlier, set your clock earlier by a small amount (e.g., 15 minutes) each morning. And similarly, plan to go to bed that much earlier each night. If you continue to get up earlier, you will become tired earlier in the evening and better able to go to sleep.

Step 2: Identify your thoughts. If you find that within an hour of your bedtime, you are still not stopping or slowing down, write down what you are doing, and what thoughts you are having about it. Use the form on the next page to record this.

For example, say you are caught up in reading the newspaper when it is time to turn out the lights and you are unable to put it down. Your thought may be, "I'll stop in a few minutes. I never get time to read the newspaper and this is really interesting."

Review your index card listing your arguments for going to bed on time, as prepared in class. Using these thoughts, write down your challange to the current (maladaptive) thought. For example, you might write, "It is more important that I get to bed. I'll really feel it tomorrow if I don't. I need to **stop right now**. I can finish reading the paper over breakfast/on the train tomorrow." This is your "counteracting thought." This is the "adaptive thought" in the form on the next page.

Step 3: Track your progress. On the last page, enter the date corresponding to the first day of each week.

Enter the time you:

1. **Actually began to get ready for bed.**
2. **Got into bed.**
3. **Fell asleep (as best you can tell the next day).**
4. **Woke up the next day, as shown.**

Continue to monitor your progress over the next month. (Remember it takes *time* to change habits.)

(cont.)

IDENTIFYING YOUR THOUGHTS

MONDAY:

Situation and thought (e.g., it's time to get ready for bed and you are sitting in front of your computer thinking, "Just a few more minutes—this YouTube video is really good.")

Adaptive thought (e.g., if I don't go to bed now, I'm going to feel tired tomorrow, and I won't be able to concentrate. I can watch the video tomorrow after work.)

TUESDAY:

Situation and thought

Adaptive thought

WEDNESDAY:

Situation and thought

Adaptive thought

(cont.)

THURSDAY:

Situation and thought

_____

Adaptive thought

_____

FRIDAY:

Situation and thought

_____

Adaptive thought

_____

SATURDAY:

Situation and thought

_____

Adaptive thought

_____

SUNDAY:

Situation and thought

_____

Adaptive thought

_____

(cont.)

TRACKING YOUR PROGRESS

Week	Date	Time preparations began	Time to bed	Time to sleep	Time wake-up (next day)
1 Monday					
Tuesday					
Wednesday					
Thursday					
Friday					
Saturday					
Sunday					
2 Monday					
Tuesday					
Wednesday					
Thursday					
Friday					
Saturday					
Sunday					
3 Monday					
Tuesday					
Wednesday					
Thursday					
Friday					
Saturday					
Sunday					
4 Monday					
Tuesday					
Wednesday					
Thursday					
Friday					
Saturday					
Sunday					

Resources

This is not intended to be a comprehensive list, but rather to highlight some resources that have come to our attention, which others with ADHD have found helpful.

PAPER PLANNERS

The following planners are all well arranged to allow for management of both schedule and to-do lists, and each includes a section for personal contact information (phone numbers, addresses, etc.). They each offer several formats, depending on how much space you need for the activities of each day: one page per day, two pages per day, two pages per week, and so on. These planners come in ring binders that allow you to insert refill sheets and easily update as needed.

FranklinCovey: *www.franklincovey.com*; 1-800-819-1812

Filofax: *www.filofaxusa.com*; 1-800-345-6798

Day Timer: *www.daytimer.com*; 1-800-225-5005

DIGITAL PLANNERS

The handheld personal digital assistant (PDA) and smartphone (BlackBerry and Android) contain software to manage one's agenda, to-do lists, and personal contacts. Information from the smartphone can be synchronized (shared) between the handheld device and a desktop or laptop computer through cable or wireless Internet access.

Two popular online planners are Google Calendar and Microsoft Outlook Calendar. They can be accessed from the smartphone that connects to the Internet anywhere, thus satisfying the "commandment" of having one's planner available at all times. These calendars can be updated via a smartphone so that the information is always current on the handheld and on multiple computers—for example, home and office.

OTHER (FREE) TASK-MANAGEMENT SOFTWARE

The following do not include calendars and thus are less ideal than integrated systems, such as those described above. However, some find these task-management functions particularly easy— even fun—to use.

ToodleDo.com

Rememberthemilk.com

RESTRICTING ACCESS TO THE INTERNET

Internet Lock helps the user to overcome the temptation to surf the Web while working on a given task. The software allows the user to password-protect access to any Internet site. Available from Toplang, *www.toplang.com/internetlock.htm.*

CONTACT MANAGEMENT

ACT! is a software program that allows the user to track contacts and manage customer relationships. Available from Sage, *www.act.com*; 1-866-873-2006.

LOGGING TIME SPENT ON COMPUTER ACTIVITIES

This software (also called a "productivity meter") allows the user to monitor how much time is spent on various predesignated computer-based activities, or online at Internet sites. Excellent for those who have to log their time (e.g., lawyers) and for others seeking to maximize their productivity. One such program is available at *www.usertime.com.* A review of various software programs available to monitor time spent online may be found at *www.smartcode.com/downloads/monitor-time-spent-online.html.* Some programs can even allocate time for you, forcing you to switch projects (by shutting down a program) when the predesignated time has expired.

MEETING PLANNING

This software automatically assembles and looks for common availability times among participants and sends out scheduling e-mails. Available free from TimeBridge, *www.TimeBridge.com.*

ASSISTANCE FOR WRITERS

- **Dragon NaturallySpeaking.** This is a voice-recognition program that allows the user to dictate directly into the computer to create text. Available from Nuance, *www.nuance.com*; 1-781-565-5000.

- **Inspiration.** This program is helpful in organizing written compositions and oral presentations. It allows the user to create a "visual map" depicting relationships among ideas and concepts, which is then easily converted into a conventional outline for text or presentation. Available from Inspiration Software, *www.inspiration.com*; 1-800-877-4292.

- **Scrivener.** This is a word processing program *for Mac OS X only*, designed for writers. Scrivener contains a metadata managing system allowing the user to keep track of notes, concepts, research, and whole documents (including text, images, audio, video, webpages, etc.) for reference. After the user has written the piece, it may be exported to a word processor such as Word for formatting. Available from Literature & Latte, *www.literatureandlatte.com/scrivener.html*.

- **Liquid Story Binder.** This program performs similar functions for Windows as Scrivener does for Mac—it allows writers to store and view their research in the same application as their writing. Available from Black Obelisk Software, *www.blackobelisksoftware.com*.

- **Page Four.** This product, for Windows, is close to Scrivener in that it expedites writing and organization for novelists and creative writers, but doesn't have the capacity to store and track the associated research. The homepage asserts, "There is no great writing, only great rewriting." Available from *www.softwareforwriting.com*.

ASSISTIVE TECHNOLOGY

- **Pulse Smartpen.** During a lecture, the audio recording and the user's notes taken with the digital pen are synchronized. Afterward, a touch of the pen at a given place in the notes activates playback of the recording at the corresponding point. Available from Livescribe, *www.Livescribe.com*; 1-877-727-4239.

- **White noise machines.** White noise machines with earphones are helpful for some in blocking out auditory distractions while working.

NATIONAL SELF-HELP GROUPS

These organizations' websites provide links to find local chapters.

Attention Deficit Disorder Association (ADDA): *www.ADD.org*.

Children and Adults with Attention Deficit/Hyperactivity Disorder (CHADD): *www.CHADD.org*.

References

Aase, H., & Sagvolden, T. (2006). Infreqeunt, but not frequent, reinforcers produce more variable responding and deficient sustained attention in young children with attention-deficit/hyperactivity disorder (ADHD). *Journal of Child Psychology and Psychiatry, 47*(5), 457–471.

Adler, L. A., Goodman, D. W., Kollins, S. H., Weisler, R. H., Krishnan, S., Zhang, Y., et al. (2008). Double-blind, placebo-controlled study of the efficacy and safety of lisdexamfetamine dimesylate in adults with attention deficit/hyperactivity disorder. *Journal of Clinical Psychiatry, 69*(9), 1364–1373.

Adler, L. A., Spencer, T., & Biederman, J. (2003). Adult ADHD Investigator Symptom Rating Scale—AISRS. Boston and New York: Massachusetts General Hospital and New York University School of Medicine.

Adler, L. A., Zimmerman, B., Starr, H. L., Silber, S., Palumbo, J., Orman, C., et al. (2009). Efficacy and safety of OROS methylphenidate in adults with attention-deficit/hyperactivity disorder: A randomized, placebo-controlled, double-blind, parallel group, dose-escalation study. *Journal of Clinical Psychopharmacology, 29*(3), 239–247.

Ainslie, G. (1974). Impulse control in pigeons. *Journal of the Experimental Analysis of Behavior, 21,* 485–489.

American Psychiatric Association. (1994). *Diagnostic and statistical manual of mental disorders* (4th ed.). Washington, DC: Author.

Applegate, B., Lahey, B. B., Hart, E. L., Biederman, J., Hynd, G. W., Barkley, R. A., et al. (1997). Validity of the age-of-onset criterion for ADHD: A report from the DSM-IV field trials. *Journal of the American Academy of Child and Adolescent Psychiatry, 36,* 1211–1221.

Barkley, R. A. (1989). The problem of stimulus control and rule-governed behavior in attention deficit disorder with hyperactivity. In L. M. Bloomingdale & J. Swanson (Eds.), *Attention deficit disorder: Current concepts and emerging trends in attentional and behavioral disorders of childhood* (pp. 203–232). Elmsford, NY: Pergamon Press.

Barkley, R. A. (1997). *ADHD and the nature of self-control.* New York: Guilford Press.

Barkley, R. A. (2006). *Attention-deficit/hyperactivity disorder: A handbook for diagnosis and treatment* (3rd ed.). New York: Guilford Press.

Barkley, R. A. (2011). *Barkley Deficits in Executive Functioning Scale (BDEFS).* New York: Guilford Press.

Barkley, R. A., & Fischer, M. (in press). Predicting impairment in major life activities in hyperactive children as adults: Self-reported executive function (EF) deficits vs. EF tests. *Developmental Neuropsychology.*

Barkley, R. A., Fischer, M., Smallish, L., & Fletcher, K. (2006). Young adult outcome of hyperactive children: Adaptive functioning in major life activities. *Journal of the American Academy of Child and Adolescent Psychiatry, 45,* 192–202.

Barkley, R. A., Koplowitz, S., Anderson, T., & McMurray, M. B. (1997). Sense of time in children with ADHD: Effects of duration, distraction, and stimulant medication. *Journal of the International Neuropsychological Society, 3,* 359–369.

Barkley, R. A., & Murphy, K. R. (1998). *Attention-deficit hyperactivity disorder: A clinical workbook.* New York: Guilford Press.

Barkley, R. A., Murphy, K. R., & Bush, T. (2001). Time perception and reproduction in young adults with attention deficit hyperactivity disorder. *Neuropsychology, 15,* 351–360.

Barkley, R. A., Murphy, K. R., & Fischer, M. (2008). *ADHD in adults: What the science says.* New York: Guilford Press.

Barkley, R. A., Murphy, K. R., O'Connell, T., & Connor, D. F. (2005). Effects of two doses of methylphenidate on simulator driving performance in adults with attention deficit hyperactivity disorder. *Journal of Safety Research, 36*(2), 121–131.

Beck, A. T., Steer, R. A., & Brown, G. K. (1996). *Manual for the Beck Depression Inventory–II* (4th ed.). San Antonio, TX: Psychological Corporation.

Beck, J. S. (1995). *Cognitive therapy: Basics and beyond.* New York: Guilford Press.

Bemporad, J. R. (2001). Aspects of psychotherapy with adults with attention deficit disorder. *Annals of the New York Academy of Sciences, 931,* 302–309.

Biederman, J., & Faraone, S. V. (2006). The effects of attention-deficit/hyperactivity disorder on employment and household income. *Medscape General Medicine, 18*(3), 12.

Biederman, J., Faraone, S. V., Spencer, J. F., Mick, E., Monuteaux, M. C., & Aleardi, M. (2006a). Functional impairments in adults with self-reports of diagnosed ADHD: A controlled study of 1001 in the community. *Journal of Clinical Psychiatry, 67*(4), 524–540.

Biederman, J., Mick, E., & Faraone, S. V. (2000). Age dependent decline of ADHD symptoms revisited: Impact of remission definition and symptom subtype. *American Journal of Psychiatry, 157,* 816–818.

Biederman, J., Mick, E., Surman, C., Doyle, R., Hammerness, P., Harpold, T., et al. (2006b). A randomized, placebo-controlled trial of OROS methylphenidate in adults with attention-deficit/hyperactivity disorder. *Biological Psychiatry, 59*(9), 829–835.

Biederman, J., Monuteaux, M. C., Doyle, A. E., Seidman, L. J., Wilens, T. E., Ferrero, F., et al. (2004). Impact of executive function deficits and attention-deficit/hyperactivity disorder (ADHD) on academic outcomes in children. *Journal of Consulting and Clinical Psychology, 72,* 757–766.

Biederman, J., Monuteaux, M. C., Mick, F., Spencer, T., Wilens, T. E., Silva, J. M., et al. (2006c).

Young adult outcome of attention deficit hyperactivity disorder: A controlled 10-year follow-up study. *Psychological Medicine, 36*(2), 167–179.

Biederman, J., Petty, C., Fried, R., Fontanella, J., Doyle, A. E., Seidman, L. J., et al. (2006d). Impact of psychometrically defined deficits of executive functioning in adults with attention deficit hyperactivity disorder. *American Journal of Psychiatry, 163*(10), 1673–1675.

Biederman, J., Petty, C. R., Monuteaux, M. C., Fried, R., Byrne, D., Mirto, T., et al. (2010). Adult psychiatric outcomes of girls with attention deficit hyperactivity disorder: 11-year follow-up in a longitudinal case-control study. *American Journal of Psychiatry, 167*(4), 409–417.

Brown, T., Reichel, P., & Quinlan, D. M. (2009). Executive function impairments in high IQ adults with ADHD. *Journal of Attention Disorders, 13*(2), 161–167.

Brown, T. E. (1996). *Attention-Deficit Disorder Scales: Manual.* San Antonio, TX: Psychological Corporation.

Brown, T. E. (2008). ADD/ADHD and impaired executive function in clinical practice. *Current Psychiatry Reports, 10*(5), 407–411.

Butler, A. C., Chapman, J. E., Forman, E. M., & Beck, A. T. (2006). The empirical status of cognitive-behavioral therapy: A review of meta-analyses. *Clinical Psychology Review, 26*(1), 17–31.

Castellanos, F. X., Sonuga-Barke, E. J., Milham, M. P., & Tannock, R. (2006). Characterizing cognition in ADHD: Beyond executive dysfunction. *Trends in Cognitive Science, 10*(3), 117–123.

Conners, C. K. (1994). *Conners' Continuous Performance Test.* Toronto: Multi-Health Systems.

Conners, C. K., Erhardt, D., & Sparrow, E. (1999). *Conners' Adult ADHD Rating Scales: Technical Manual.* Toronto: Multi-Health Systems.

Douglas, V. I. (1999). Cognitive control processes in attention-deficit/hyperactivity disorder. In H. C. Quay & A. E. Hogan (Eds.), *Handbook of disruptive behavior disorders* (pp. 105–138). New York: Kluwer Academic/Plenum.

Doyle, A. E. (2006). Executive functions in attention-deficit/hyperactivity disorder. *Journal of Clinical Psychiatry, 67*(Suppl 8), 21–26.

Epstein, J. N., Johnson, D. E., & Conners, C. K. (2001). *Conners' Adult ADHD Diagnostic Interview for DSM-IV.* North Tonawanda, NY: Multi-Health Systems.

Faraone, S. V., Biederman, J., Weber, W., & Russell, R. L. (1998). Psychiatric, neuropsychological, and psychosocial features of DSM-IV subtypes of attention-deficit/hyperactivity disorder: Results from a clinically referred sample. *Journal of the American Academy of Child and Adolescent Psychiatry, 37,* 185–193.

Faraone, S. V., & Glatt, S. J. (2010). A comparison of the efficacy of medications for adult attention-deficit/hyperactivity disorder using meta-analysis of effect sizes. *Journal of Clinical Psychiatry, 71*(6), 754–763.

First, M. B., Gibbon, M., Spitzer, R. L., Williams, J. B. W., & Benjamin, L. S. (1997). *Structured Clinical Interview for DSM-IV Axis II Personality Disorders (SCID-II).* Washington, DC: American Psychiatric Press.

First, M. B., Spitzer, R. L., Gibbon, M., & Williams, J. B. W. (2002). *Structured Clinical Interview for DSM-IV-TR Axis I Disorders—Patient Edition (SCID-I/P, 11/2002 rev.).* New York: Biometrics Research Department, New York State Psychiatric Institute.

Goodwin, R. E., & Corgiat, M. D. (1992). Cognitive rehabilitation of adult attention deficit disorder: A case study. *Journal of Cognitive Rehabilitation, 10*(5), 28–35.

Haenlein, M., & Caul, W. (1987). Attention deficit disorder with hyperactivity: A specific hypothesis of reward dysfunction. *Journal of the American Academy of Child and Adolescent Psychiatry, 26*, 356–362.

Hervey, A. S., Epstein, J. N., & Curry, J. F. (2004). Neuropsychology of adults with attention-deficit/hyperactivity disorder: A meta-analytic review. *Neuropsychology, 18*(3), 485–503.

Hesslinger, B., Tebartz van Elst, L., Nyberg, E., Dykierek, P., Richter, H., Berner, M., et al. (2002). Psychotherapy of attention deficit hyperactivity disorder in adults—A pilot study using a structured skills training program. *European Archives of Psychiatry and Clinical Neuroscience, 252*, 177–184.

Kessler, R. C., Adler, L. A., Barkley, R. A., Biederman, J., Conners, C. K., Demler, O., et al. (2006). The prevalence and correlates of adult ADHD in the United States: Results from the national comorbidity survey replication. *American Journal of Psychiatry, 163*, 716–723.

Lahey, B. B., Pelham, W. E., Loney, J., Lee, S. S., & Willcutt, E. (2005). Instability of the DSM-IV subtypes of ADHD from preschool through elementary school. *Archives of General Psychiatry, 62*(8), 896–902.

Leark, P. A., Greenberg, L. K., Kindschi, C. L., Dupuy, T. R., & Hughes, S. J. (2007). *Test of Variables of Attention: Clinical manual.* Los Alamitos, CA: TOVA.

Luman, M., Oosterlaan, J., & Sergeant, J. A. (2005). The impact of reinforcement contingencies on AD/HD: A review and theoretical appraisal. *Clinical Psychology Review, 25*(2), 183–213.

Mannuzza, S., Klein, R. G., Bessler, A., Malloy, P., & LaPadula, M. (1998). Adult psychiatric status of hyperactive boys grown up. *American Journal of Psychiatry, 155*, 493–498.

McBurnett, K., Pfiffner, L. J., Willcutt, E., Tamm, L., Lerner, M., Ottolini, Y. L., et al. (1999). Experimental cross-validation of DSM-IV types of attention-deficit/hyperactivity disorder. *Journal of the American Academy of Child and Adolescent Psychiatry, 38*, 17–24.

McDermott, S. P., & Wilens, T. E. (2000). Cognitive therapy for adults with ADHD. In T. Brown (Ed.), *Attention deficit disorders and comorbidities in children, adolescents, and adults* (pp. 569–606). Washington, DC: American Psychiatric Press.

Medori, R., Ramos-Quiroga, A., Casas, M., Kooij, J. J. S., Niemela, A., Trott, G.-E., et al. (2008). A randomized, placebo-controlled trial of three fixed dosages of prolonged-release OROS methylphenidate in adults with attention-deficit/hyperactivity disorder. *Biological Psychiatry, 63*, 981–989.

Michelson, D., Adler, L., Spencer, T., Reimherr, F. W., West, S. A., Allen, A. J., et al. (2003). Atomoxetine in adults with ADHD: Two randomized, placebo-controlled studies. *Biological Psychiatry, 53*(2), 112–120.

Morgenstern, J. (2004). *Organizing from the inside out: The foolproof system for organizing your home, your office, and your life.* New York: Holt.

Nigg, J. T. (2006). *What causes ADHD?: Understanding what goes wrong and why.* New York: Guilford Press.

Prochaska, J. O., & Norcross, J. C. (2001). Stages of change. *Psychotherapy, 38*, 443–448.

Quinlan, D. M., & Brown, T. E. (2003). Assessment of short-term verbal memory impairments in adolescents and adults with ADHD. *Journal of Attention Disorders, 6*(4), 143–152.

Ramsay, J. R., & Rostain, A. L. (2008). *Cognitive-behavioral therapy for adult ADHD: An integrative psychosocial and medical approach.* New York: Routledge.

Riccio, C. A., & Reynolds, C. R. (2001). Continuous performance tests are sensitive to ADHD in adults but lack specificity. A review and critique for differential diagnosis. *Annals of the New York Academy of Science, 931*, 113–139.

Rosenberg, M. (1965). *Society and the adolescent self-image.* Princeton, NJ: Princeton University Press.

Rostain, A. L., & Ramsay, J. R. (2006). A combined treatment approach for adults with ADHD—Results of an open study of 43 patients. *Journal of Attention Disorders, 10*(2), 150–159.

Roth, R. M., Isquith, P. K., & Gioia, G. A. (2005). *Behavior Rating Inventory of Executive Function—Adult Version (BRIEF-A).* Lutz, FL: Psychological Assessment Resources.

Safren, S. A., Otto, M. W., Sprich, S., Winett, C. L., Wilens, T. E., & Biederman, J. J. (2005). Cognitive-behavioral therapy for ADHD in medication-treated adults with continued symptoms. *Behaviour Research and Therapy, 43*(7), 831–842.

Safren, S. A., Sprich, S., Mimiaga, M. J., Surman, C., Knouse, L., et al. (2010). Cognitive-behavioral therapy vs. relaxation with educational support for medication-treated adults with ADHD and persistent symptoms: A randomized controlled trial. *Journal of the American Medical Association, 304*(8), 875–880.

Sanford, J. A., & Turner, A. (2004). *The Integrated Visual and Auditory Continuous Performance Test. Interpretive manual.* Richmond, VA: BrainTrain.

Seidman, L. J., Valera, E. M., & Bush, G. (2004). Brain function and structure in adults with attention-deficit/hyperactivity disorder. *Psychiatric Clinics of North America, 27*(2), 323–347.

Seidman, L. J., Valera, E. M., & Makris, N. (2005). Structural brain imaging of attention-deficit/hyperactivity disorder. *Biological Psychiatry, 57*(11), 1263–1272.

Seligman, M. E. P. (1975). *Helplessness: On depression, development, and death.* New York: Freeman.

Semrud-Clikeman, M., Biederman, J., Sprich-Buckminster, S., Lehman, B. K., Faraone, S. V., & Norman, D. (1992). Comorbidity between ADDH and learning disability: A review and report in a clinically referred sample. *Journal of the American Academy of Child and Adolescent Psychiatry, 31*, 439–448.

Sergeant, J. A. (2005). Modeling attention-deficit/hyperactivity disorder: A critical appraisal of the cognitive-energetic model. *Biological Psychiatry, 57*(11), 1248–1255.

Shear, M. K., Vanderbilt, J., Rucci, P., Endicott, J., Lydiard, B., Otto, M. W., et al. (2001). Reliability and validity of a structured interview guide for the Hamilton Anxiety Rating Scale (SIGH-A). *Depression and Anxiety, 13*, 166–178.

Smalley, S. L., McGough, J. J., Del'Homme, M., NewDelman, J., Gordon, E., Ki Liu, A., et al. (2000). Familial clustering of symptoms and disruptive behaviors in multiplex families with attention-deficit/hyperactivity disorder. *Journal of the American Academy of Child and Adolescent Psychiatry, 39*, 1135–1143.

Solanto, M. V., Etefia, K., & Marks, D. J. (2004). The utility of self-report measures and the Continuous Performance Test in the diagnosis of ADHD in adults. *CNS Spectrums, 9*, 649–659.

Solanto, M. V., Gilbert, S. N., Raj, A., Zhu, J., Pope-Boyd, S., Stepak, B., et al. (2007). Neurocognitive functioning in ADHD, predominantly inattentive subtype. *Journal of Abnormal Child Psychology, 35*(5), 729–744.

Solanto, M. V., Marks, D. J., Mitchell, K., Wasserstein, J., & Kofman, M. D. (2008). Development of a new psychosocial treatment for adults with ADHD. *Journal of Attention Disorders, 11*(6), 728–736.

Solanto, M. V., Marks, D. J., Wasserstein, J., Mitchell, K., Abikoff, H., Alvir, J. M., et al. (2010). Efficacy of meta-cognitive therapy for adult ADHD. *American Journal of Psychiatry, 167*(8), 958–968.

Sonuga-Barke, E. J. S. (2003). The dual pathway model of AD/HD: An elaboration of neuro-developmental characteristics. *Neuroscience and Biobehavioral Reviews, 27,* 593–604.

Sonuga-Barke, E. J., Sergeant, J. A., Nigg, J., & Willcutt, E. (2008). Executive dysfunction and delay aversion in attention deficit hyperactivity disorder: Nosologic and diagnostic implications. *Child and Adolescent Psychiatric Clinics of North America, 17*(2), 367–384.

Spencer, T., Biederman, J., & Wilens, T. (2004a). Nonstimulant treatment of adult attention-deficit/hyperactivity disorder. *Psychiatric Clinics of North America, 27*(2), 373–383.

Spencer, T., Biederman, J., & Wilens, T. (2004b). Stimulant treatment of adult attention-deficit/hyperactivity disorder. *Psychiatric Clinics of North America, 27*(2), 361–372.

Spencer, T., Biederman, J., Wilens, T., Doyle, R., Surman, C., Prince, J., et al. (2005). A large, double-blind, randomized clinical trial of methylphenidate in the treatment of adults with attention-deficit/hyperactivity disorder. *Biological Psychiatry, 57*(5), 456–463.

Spencer, T., Biederman, J., Wilens, T., Faraone, S., Prince, J., Girard, K., et al. (2001). Efficacy of a mixed amphetamine salts compound in adults with ADHD. *Archives of General Psychiatry, 58,* 775–782.

Stevenson, C. S., Whitmont, S., Bornholt, L., Livesey, D., & Stevenson, R. J. (2002). A cognitive remediation programme for adults with attention deficit hyperactivity disorder. *Australian and New Zealand Journal of Psychiatry, 36,* 610.

Tellegen, A., & Briggs, P. F. (1967). Old wine, new skins: Grouping Wechsler subtests into new scales. *Journal of Consulting and Clinical Psychology, 31*(5), 499–506.

Tucker, D. M., & Williamson, P. A. (1984). Asymmetric neural control systems in human self-regulation. *Psychological Review, 91,* 185–215.

Virta, M., Vedenpaa, A., Gronroos, N., Chydenius, E., Partinen, M., Vataja, R., et al. (2008). Adults with ADHD benefit from cognitive-behaviorally oriented group rehabilitation: A study of 29 participants. *Journal of Attention Disorders, 12*(3), 218–226.

Wasserstein, J., & Denckla, M. B. (2009). ADHD and learning disabilities in ADHD: Overlap with executive dysfunction. In T. E. Brown (Ed.), *ADHD comorbidities: Handbook for ADHD complications in children and adults* (pp. 233–247). Arlington, VA: American Psychiatric Publishing.

Wasserstein, J., & Lynn, A. (2001). Metacognitive remediation in adult ADHD: Treating executive function deficits via executive functions. *Annals of the New York Academy of Science, 931,* 376–384.

Wasserstein, J., Wolf, L. E., Solanto, M., Marks, D., & Simkowitz, P. (2008). Adult attention deficit hyperactivity disorder: Basic and clinical issues. In J. F. Morgan & J. H. Ricker (Eds.), *Handbook of clinical neuropsychology* (pp. 679–695). Lisse, The Netherlands: Swets & Zeitlinger.

Weisler, R. H., Biederman, J., Spencer, T. J., Wilens, T. E., Faraone, S. V., Chrisman, A. K., et al. (2006). Mixed amphetamine salts extended-release in the treatment of adult ADHD: A randomized, controlled trial. *CNS Spectrums, 11*(8), 625–639.

Weiss, G., & Hechtman, L. (1993). *Hyperactive children grown up: Empirical findings and theoretical considerations* (2nd ed.). New York: Guilford Press.

Wiggins, D., Singh, K., Getz, H., & Hutchins, D. (1999). Effects of a brief group intervention for adults with attention-deficit/hyperactivity disorder. *Journal of Mental Health Counseling, 21,* 82–92.

Wilens, T. E. (2008). Pharmacotherapy of ADHD in adults. *CNS Spectrums, 13*(5 Suppl 8), 11–13.

Wilens, T. E., McDermott, S., Biederman, J., Abrantes, A., Hahesy, A., & Spencer, T. (1999). Cognitive therapy in the treatment of adults with ADHD: A systematic chart review of 26 cases. *Journal of Cognitive Psychotherapy: An International Quarterly, 13,* 215–226.

Willcutt, E. G., Doyle, A. E., Nigg, J. T., Faraone, S. V., & Pennington, B. F. (2005). Validity of the executive function theory of attention-deficit/hyperactivity disorder: A meta-analytic review. *Biological Psychiatry, 57*(11), 1336–1346.

Wolraich, M. L., Hannah, J. N., Pinnock, T. Y., Baumgaertel, A., & Brown, J. (1996). Comparison of diagnostic criteria for attention-deficit hyperactivity disorder in a county-wide sample. *Journal of the American Academy of Child and Adolescent Psychiatry, 35,* 319–324.

Index